# CLINICAL ETHICS

## NOTICE

Medicine is an ever-changing science. As new research and clinical experience broaden our knowledge, changes in treatment and drug therapy are required. The authors and the publisher of this work have checked with sources believed to be reliable in their efforts to provide information that is complete and generally in accord with the standards accepted at the time of publication. However, in view of the possibility of human error or changes in medical sciences, neither the authors nor the publisher nor any other party who has been involved in the preparation or publication of this work warrants that the information contained herein is in every respect accurate or complete, and they are not responsible for any errors or omissions or for the results obtained from use of such information. Readers are encouraged to confirm the information contained herein with other sources. For example and in particular, readers are advised to check the product information sheet included in the package of each drug they plan to administer to be certain that the information contained in this book is accurate and that changes have not been made in the recommended dose or in the contraindications for administration. This recommendation is of particular importance in connection with new or infrequently used drugs.

FOURTH EDITION

# CLINICAL ETHICS

## A Practical Approach to Ethical Decisions in Clinical Medicine

### Albert R. Jonsen, Ph.D.

Professor of Ethics in Medicine
Chairman, Department of Medical History and Ethics
University of Washington School of Medicine
Seattle, Washington

### Mark Siegler, M.D.

Lindy Bergman Professor of Medicine
Director, MacLean Center for Clinical Medical Ethics
University of Chicago
Chicago, Illinois

### William J. Winslade, Ph.D., J.D.

James Wade Rockwell Professor of Philosophy of Medicine
Institute for the Medical Humanities
Director, Ethics Consultation Service
University of Texas Medical Branch at Galveston
Galveston, Texas

## McGraw-Hill
## Health Professions Division

New York · St. Louis · San Francisco · Auckland · Bogotá
Caracas · Lisbon · London · Madrid · Mexico City · Milan · Montreal
New Delhi · San Juan · Singapore · Sydney · Tokyo · Toronto

# McGraw-Hill

A Division of The **McGraw·Hill** Companies

**Clinical Ethics: A Practical Approach to Ethical Decisions in Clinical Medicine, Fourth Edition**

Copyright © 1998, 1992, 1986, 1982 by The McGraw-Hill Companies, Inc.

1 2 3 4 5 6 7 8 9 0 DOC DOC 9 9 8 7

ISBN 0-07-033120-0

This book was set in Garamond Book by V&M Graphics, Inc.
The editors were John Dolan and P. McCurdy;
the production supervisor was Heather Munro;
the designer was Robert Freese;
R.R. Donnelley and Sons was printer and binder.

This book is printed on acid-free paper.

Cataloging-in-Publication Data is on file for this title at the Library of Congress.

# Contents

# Locator

**Boldface numbers** indicate major discussions of the topic.

# CLINICAL ETHICS

# Introduction

## CASE ANALYSIS IN CLINICAL ETHICS

Clinical ethics is a practical discipline that provides a structured approach to assist physicians in identifying, analyzing, and resolving ethical issues in clinical medicine. The practice of good clinical medicine requires some working knowledge about ethical issues such as informed consent, truth-telling, confidentiality, end-of-life care, pain relief, and patient rights. Medicine, even at its most technical and scientific, is an encounter between human beings, and the physician's work of diagnosing disease, offering advice, and providing treatment is embedded in a moral context. Usually, values such as mutual respect, honesty, trustworthiness, compassion, and a commitment to pursue shared goals make a clinical encounter between physician and patient morally unproblematic. Occasionally, physicians and patients may disagree about values or face choices that challenge their values. It is then that ethical problems arise. Clinical ethics is both about the ethical features that are present in every clinical encounter and about the ethical problems that occasionally arise in those encounters. Clinical ethics relies upon the conviction that, even when perplexity is great and emotions run high, physicians and nurses, patients and families can work constructively to identify, analyze, and resolve many of the ethical problems that arise in clinical medicine.

We have two purposes in writing this book: first, to offer an approach that facilitates thinking about the complexities of the problems that clinicians actually face and, second, to assemble concise representative opinions about typical ethical problems that occur in the practice of medicine. We think it is more important that clinicians develop skill at analyzing the cases they encounter rather than merely have a book in which "to look up answers." Our hope is that every clinician will acknowledge that ethics is an inherent aspect of good clinical medicine and that, ideally, every clinician will become as proficient at clinical ethics as at clinical medicine. Our book is intended not only for clinicians and students who provide care to patients, but also for others whose work requires an awareness and sensitivity to the ethical issues raised in clinical care, such as hospital chaplains administrators, hospital attorneys, members of institutional ethics committees, quality reviewers, and administrators of health plans. In the complex world of modern health care, all of these persons are responsible for maintaining the ethics that lie at the heart of quality care.

Many books on health care ethics are organized around moral principles, such as respect for autonomy, beneficence, nonmaleficence and fairness, and the cases are analyzed in the light of those principles. Our method is different. While we appreciate the importance of principles, we believe that the practitioner approaching a case needs a method that better fits the realities of the clinical setting. Clinical situations are complex since they often involve a wide range of medical facts, a multitude of circumstances, and a variety of values. Often decisions must be reached quickly. The authors believe that clinicians need a straightforward way to sort the facts and values of the case at hand into an orderly pattern that will facilitate the discussion and resolution of the ethical problem.

We suggest that every clinical case, when seen as an ethical problem, should be analyzed by means of four topics. These four topics are (1) medical indications, (2) patient preferences, (3) quality of life, and (4) contextual features, that is, the social, economic, legal, and administrative context in which the case occurs. Every case can be viewed in terms of these four topics; no case can be adequately discussed without reference to them. Although the facts of each case differ, these four topics are always relevant. The topics organize the varying facts of the particular case and, at the same time, the topics call attention to the moral principles appropriate to the case. It is our intent to show readers how the topics provide a systematic way to identify, analyze, and resolve the ethical problems arising in clinical medicine.

Clinicians will recall the method of case presentation that they learned at the beginning of their professional training. They were taught to "present" a patient by stating in order the patient's chief complaint, the history of the present illness, past medical history, family and social history, followed by physical findings and laboratory data. These are the topics that an experienced clinician uses to reach a diagnosis and to formulate a case management plan. While the particular details under each of these topics differ from patient to patient, the topics themselves are constant and always relevant to the task of arriving at a case management plan. Sometimes one topic—for example, the patient's family history or the physical examination—may be particularly important or, conversely, may not be relevant to the problem at hand. Still, clinicians are expected to review all topics in every case. Our four topics—(1) medical indications, (2) patient preferences, (3) quality of life, and (4) contextual features—are the ethical equivalents of these familiar clinical topics.

These topics help clinicians understand where the moral principles meet the circumstances of the clinical case. The general headings under the topics describe the major features that define the ethics of clinical medicine; each of these features takes on specific, concrete form from the circumstances of the particular case. In a given case, a patient comes to a physician, complaining of feeling ill. Medical indications include a clinical picture of polydipsia and polyuria, nausea, fatigue, and some mental confusion, with laboratory studies showing hyperglycemia, acidosis, and elevated plasma ketone concentrations. A diagnosis of diabetic ketoacidosis is made. Fluids and insulin are indicated in specific doses and volumes. These particulars are the occasion for implementing the moral principle of beneficence, that is, the duty of performing actions that benefit the patient. However, in the same case, the patient may be confused and, after hearing the physician's recommendations, rejects further medical attention. These circumstances, noted under Patient Preferences, raise questions about the principle of autonomy, that is, the duty to respect the patient's wishes. As the case is described, circumstances accumulate under all four of the topics and affect the meaning and relevance of the moral principles. It is advisable to review the entire four topics in order to see how the principles and the circumstances together define the ethical problem in the case and suggest a resolution. It is rare that an ethical problem involves only one ethical principle. Every actual ethical problem is a complex collection of many circumstances. Good ethical judgment consists in appreciating how several ethical principles should be evaluated in the actual situation under consideration. We hope our method helps practitioners to do just that.

We divide the book into four chapters, each one devoted to one of these four topics. These four chapters define the major concepts associated with each topic, present typical cases in which the topic under discussion plays a particularly important role, and critically review the arguments commonly offered to resolve the problem. For example, the case of a Jehovah's Witness patient who refuses blood transfusion will demonstrate how the topic of patient preferences functions in the analysis of the ethical problem raised by a patient's refusal of an indicated medical treatment. At the same time, the current opinion of medical ethicists on Jehovah's Witness cases will be summarized. Thus, a reader can use this volume as a reference book, looking up, for example, "refusal of treatment" or "Jehovah's Witnesses" in the Locator at the front of the book and reading the several pages devoted to that issue in Chapter 2.

Those who use the book as a reference will find concise summaries of current opinion on the ethics of certain typical cases, such as those involving refusal of care or a diagnosis of persistent vegetative state. This may be all that they seek at the moment. However, the actual cases that clinicians encounter in practice will be more than typical: they will be a combination of unique circumstances and values. The four topics are, as it were, signposts that guide the way through the complexity of real cases. Thus, mastering the book's four-part method will serve the reader better than using it for occasional reference. We strongly suggest that readers first read the book from beginning to end to get the hang of the method. We hope they will become adept at bringing the method to bear on their own clinical cases.

This book was originally written for physicians specialized in internal medicine and concentrated on the ethical problems encountered by those making clinical decisions for patients in their practice. In subsequent editions, the scope was broadened to adult medicine in general and then to pediatrics. (The sections particularly relevant to pediatric ethics have **P** after their numbers in the text.) It also became obvious to the authors that many other health care providers, nurses, social workers, medical technicians, as well as chaplains and administrators, found our method useful. In this fourth edition, the original emphasis on clinical decisions made by physicians remains, but we believe that others can fit the particular concerns and values of their own professions into the topics of the book.

We illustrate our method by a brief summary of a case familiar to many who have studied medical ethics, namely, the case of Donald "Dax" Cowart, the burn patient who related his experience in the videotape *Please Let Me Die* and the documentary *Dax's Case*.[1]

In 1973, "Dax" Cowart, age 25, was severely burned in a propane gas explosion. Rushed to the Burn Treatment Unit of Parkland Hospital in Dallas, he was found to have severe burns over 65 percent of his body; his face and hands suffered third degree burns and his eyes were severely damaged. Full burn therapy was instituted. After an initial period during which his survival was in doubt, he stabilized and underwent amputation of several fingers and removal of his right eye. During much of his 232 day hospitalization at Parkland, his few weeks at Texas Institute of Rehabilitation and Research at Houston, and his subsequent six months' stay at University of Texas Medical Branch in Galveston, he repeatedly insisted that treatment be discontinued and that he be allowed to die. Despite this demand, wound care was continued, skin grafts performed and nutritional and fluid support provided. He was discharged totally blind, with minimal use of his hands, badly scarred, and dependent on others to assist in personal functions.

Discussion of a case like this can begin by raising any number of questions. Did Dax have the moral or the legal right to refuse care? Was Dax competent to make a decision? Were the physicians paternalistic? What was Dax's prognosis? All these questions, and many others, are relevant and can give rise to vigorous debate. However, we suggest that an ethical analysis should begin with an orderly review of the four topics. We recommend that the same order be followed in all cases: (1) medical indications, (2) patient preferences, (3) quality of life, (4) contextual features. This procedure will lay out the ethically relevant facts of the case (or show where further information is needed) before debate begins. It should be noted that this order of review does not constitute an order of ethical priority. The determination of relative importance of these topics will be explained in the four chapters.

**Medical Indications.** This topic comprises the usual content of a clinical discussion: the diagnosis and treatment of the patient's pathological condition. "Indications" refers to the relation between the pathophysiology presented by the patient and the diagnostic and therapeutic interventions that are "indicated," that is, appropriate to evaluate and treat the problem. Although this is the usual material covered in the presentation of any patient's clinical problems, the ethical discussion will not only review the medical facts but also attend to the purposes and goals of any indicated interventions.

In Dax's case, the medical indications include the clinical facts necessary to diagnose the extent and seriousness of burns, to make a prognosis for survival or restoration of function, and to select among the options for treatment, including the risks, benefits and probable outcomes of each treatment modality. For example, certain prognoses are associated with burns of given severity and extent. Various forms of treatment, such as fluid replacement, skin grafting, and antibiotics, are associated with certain probabilities of outcome and risk. After initial emergency treatment, Dax's prognosis for survival was approximately 20 percent. After six months of intensive care, his prognosis for survival improved to almost 100 percent. If his request to stop wound care and grafting during that hospitalization had been respected, he would almost certainly have died. A clear view of the possible benefits of intervention is the first step in assessing the ethical aspects of a case.

**Patient Preferences.** In all medical treatment, the preferences of the patient, based on the patient's own values and personal assessment of benefits and burdens, are ethically relevant. In every clinical case, the questions must be raised: "What are the patient's goals? What does the patient want?" The systematic review of this topic requires further questions. Has the patient been provided sufficient information? Does the patient comprehend? Does the patient understand the uncertainty inherent in any medical recommendation and the range of reasonable options that exist? Is the patient consenting voluntarily? Is the patient coerced? In some cases, an answer to these questions might be "We don't know because the patient is incapable of formulating a preference or expressing one." If the patient is mentally incapacitated at the time a decision must be made, we must ask, "Who has the authority to decide on behalf of this patient? What are the ethical and legal limits of that authority? What is to be done if no one can be identified as surrogate?"

In Dax's case, a question about his mental capacity arose in the early days of his refusal of care. Had the physical and emotional shock of the accident undermined his ability to decide for himself? Initially it was assumed that he lacked the capacity to make his own decisions, at least about refusing lifesaving therapy. The doctors accepted the consent of Dax's mother in favor of treatment, over his refusal of treatment. Later, when Dax was hospitalized in Galveston, psychiatric consultation was requested which affirmed his capacity to make decisions. Once capacity was established, the ethical implications of his desire to refuse care became central. Should his preference be respected? If not, on what grounds? Did Dax appreciate sufficiently the prospects for his rehabilitation? Are physicians obliged to pursue therapies they believe have promise over the objections of a patient? Would they be cooperating in a suicide if they assented to Dax's wishes? Any case involving the ethics of patient preferences relies on clarification of these questions.

**Quality of Life.**   Any injury or illness threatens persons with actual or potential reduced quality of life, manifested in the signs and symptoms of their disease. The object of all medical intervention is to restore, maintain, or improve quality of life. Thus, in all medical situations, the topic of quality of life must be raised. Many questions surround this topic: What does this phrase, "quality of life," mean in general? How should it be understood in particular cases? How do persons other than the patient perceive the patient's quality of life and of what ethical relevance are their perceptions? Above all, what is the relevance of quality of life to ethical judgment? This topic, which is less well worked out in the literature of medical ethics than the two previous ones, is perilous because it opens the door for bias and prejudice. Still, it must be confronted in the analysis of clinical ethical problems.

In Dax's case, we note the quality of his life prior to the accident. He was a popular, athletic young man, just discharged from the Air Force, after serving as a fighter pilot in Viet Nam. He worked in a real estate business with his father (who was also injured in the explosion and died on the way to the hospital). Before his accident, Dax's quality of life was excellent. During the course of medical care, he endured excruciating pain and profound depression. After the accident, even with the best of care, he was confronted with significant physical deficits, including notable disfigurement, blindness, and limitation of activity. At some stage in his illness, Dax had the capacity to determine what quality of life he wished for himself. However, in the early weeks of his hospitalization, he was probably mentally incapacitated at the time critical decisions had to be made. When he was, others would have had to make certain quality-of-life decisions on his behalf. Was the prospect for return to a normal or even acceptable life so poor that no reasonable person would choose to live? Who should make such decisions? What values should guide them? The meaning and import of such considerations must be clarified in any clinical ethical analysis.

**Contextual Features.**    Patients come to physicians because they have a problem that they hope the physician can help to correct. Physicians undertake the care of patients with the intent and the duty to make all reasonable efforts to help them. The topics of medical indications, patient preferences, and quality of life bring out these essential features of the case. Yet every medical case is embedded in a larger context of persons, institutions, financial and social arrangements. Patient care is influenced, positively or negatively, by the possibilities and the constraints of that context. At the same time, the context itself is affected by the decisions made by or about the patient: these decisions have psychological, emotional, financial, legal, scientific, educational, religious impact on others. In every case, the relevance of the contextual features must be determined and assessed. These contextual features may be crucially important to the understanding and resolution of the case.

In Dax's case, several of these contextual features were significant. Dax's mother was opposed to termination of medical care for religious reasons. The legal implications of honoring Dax's demand were unclear at the time. (They are clearer today.) The costs of sixteen months of intensive burn therapy are not insignificant (although this was not emphasized in the various discussions of the case). The distress caused to medical and nursing personnel by Dax's refusal to cooperate with treatment might have influenced their attitudes toward him. These and other contextual factors must be made explicit and assessed for their relevance.

These four topics are relevant to any clinical case, whatever the actual circumstances. They serve as a useful organizing device for teaching and discussion. More important, however, is the way in which a review of these topics can help to move a discussion of an ethical problem toward a resolution. Any serious discussion of an ethical problem must go beyond merely talking about it in an orderly way: it must push through to a reasonable and practical resolution. Ethical problems, no less than medical problems, cannot be left hanging. Thus, after presenting a case, the task of seeking a resolution must begin.

The discussion of each topic raises, or presupposes, certain common ethical notions. These notions propose certain standards of behavior or attitudes that are morally appropriate to the topic. They can be called moral principles or rules: rules tend to be quite specific to particular topics, while principles are stated in broader, more general terms. For example, one version of the principle of beneficence states, "There is an obligation to assist others in serious need." The moral rule, "Physicians have a duty to treat patients, even at risk to themselves," is a specific expression of that broad principle, suited to a particular sphere of professional activity, namely, medical care. The topic of medical indications, in addition to the clinical data that must be discussed, raises the further questions, "How much can we do to help this patient?" "What risks of adverse effects can be tolerated in the attempt to treat the patient?" Answers to these questions, arising so naturally in the discussion of medical indications, can be guided by familiar moral rules applied to medical ethics such as, "Be of benefit and do no harm," or "Risks should be balanced by benefits." Rules such as these reflect in a specific way the broad principle that the philosophers have named beneficence. Similarly, the topic of patient preferences contains rules that instruct clinicians to tell patients the truth, to respect their deliberate preferences, to honor their values, etc. Rules such as these fall under the general scope of the principles of autonomy and respect for persons.

Our method of analysis begins, not with the principles and rules, as do many other ethics treatises, but with the factual features of the case. We refer to relevant principles and rules as they arise in the discussion of the topics. In this way, abstract discussion of principles is avoided as is the tendency to think of only one principle, such as autonomy or beneficence, as the sole guide in the case. Moral rules and principles are best appreciated in the specific context of the actual circumstances of a case. For example, a key issue in Dax's case is the autonomy of the patient. However, the significance of autonomy in Dax's case is derived, not simply from the principle that requires we respect it, but from the confluence of considerations about preferences, medical indications for treatment, quality of life, decisional capacity, and the roles of his mother, the doctors, the lawyers, and the hospitals. Only when all these are seen and evaluated in relation to each other will the meaning of the principle of autonomy be appreciated in this case.

Competence in clinical ethics depends not only on being able to use a sound method for analysis but also on familiarity with the literature of medical ethics. Some readers will seek further elaboration of the issues dealt with so briefly in this introductory book. We direct these readers to a few sources where they will find not only that elaboration but references to the major literature. Thus, we place in brackets after our discussion of an issue references to *The Encyclopedia of Bioethics*,[2] *Principles of Biomedical Ethics*,[3] and *Medical Ethics*.[4] These books will be abbreviated as EB, PBE, ME. We note a few books or special issues of journals that provide ample treatment of a particular topic. We rarely cite articles: the literature in medical ethics that appears in medical and bioethical journals is extensive and much of it becomes rapidly outdated. We will, of course, cite those articles that we quote and also the occasional review article that can introduce readers to a broader discussion. Readers seeking the most current articles may search in the annual publication *Bibliography of Bioethics*.[5] This source is available online as Bioethicsline, through the National Library of Medicine's MEDLARS. At the end of the book, we list the major resources for further study in bioethics.

## FOUR CASES

Four clinical cases will reappear throughout this book as our major examples. The patients in these cases are given the names Mr. Cure, Mr. Cope, Mrs. Care, and Ms. Comfort. These fictional names are chosen to suggest certain prominent features of their medical condition. Mr. Cure suffers from bacterial meningitis, a serious, but curable, acute condition. Mr. Cope has a chronic condition, insulin-dependent diabetes, that requires certain medical assistance but depends heavily on the patient's active involvement in his own care. Mrs. Care has multiple sclerosis, a disease that cannot be cured but whose inexorable deterioration can be managed by continual care. Ms. Comfort has breast cancer that has metastasized, for which there is a low probability of cure even under a regimen of intensive intervention. Details of these cases will occasionally be changed to illustrate various points as the text proceeds. Many other shorter case examples will appear in which the patients will be designated by initials.

**Case I.** Mr. Cure, a 24-year-old white male, has been brought to the emergency room by a friend. Previously in good health, he is complaining of severe headache and a stiff neck. The results of the physical examination and laboratory studies, including spinal fluid examination, suggest a diagnosis of pneumococcal pneumonia and pneumococcal meningitis.

**Case II.** Mr. Cope is a 42-year-old man with insulin-dependent diabetes. His diabetes was first diagnosed at age 21. He complied with an insulin and dietary regimen quite faithfully. Still, he experienced frequent episodes of ketoacidosis and hypoglycemia, which necessitated repeated hospitalizations and emergency room care. For the past few years, his diabetes has been controlled, and he required hospitalization only once for ketoacidosis associated with acute pyelonephritis. Twenty-one years after the onset of diabetes, he appears to have no functional impairment from his disease. However, funduscopic examination reveals a moderate number of microaneurysms, and urinalysis shows persistent proteinuria. He has no neurological symptoms or abnormal physical findings.

**Case III.** Mrs. Care, a 48-year-old married woman with two children, was diagnosed with multiple sclerosis (MS) 15 years ago. Over the past 12 years, the patient has experienced progressive deterioration. She developed severe spasticity in both legs, requiring canes, then a walker, and finally full use of a wheelchair. She is now blind in one eye, with markedly decreased vision in the other. For the past two years, she has required an indwelling Foley catheter due to an atonic bladder. In the last year, she has become profoundly depressed, uncommunicative even with close family, and refuses to rise from bed.

**Case IV.** Ms. Comfort is a 58-year-old woman. She has had a mammogram yearly for the past six years. Eight months after her last mammogram, she noted a rapidly increasing right breast mass. She was seen by her primary care physician and referred to a surgeon who performed a breast biopsy that confirmed the presence of an infiltrating ductal adenocarcinoma. She underwent a modified radical mastectomy with reconstruction. Dissected nodes revealed metastatic disease. She received a course of chemotherapy and radiation, with tamoxifen.

## References

1. Kliever LD, ed. *Dax's Case. Essays in Medical Ethics and Human Meaning*. Dallas: Southern Methodist University Press, 1989.
2. Reich W, ed. *Encyclopedia of Bioethics*. 2nd edition. 5 vols. New York: Simon & Schuster/Macmillan, 1995.
3. Beauchamp TL, Childress JF. *Principles of Biomedical Ethics*. New York: Oxford University Press, 4th edition, 1994.
4. Veatch RM, ed. *Medical Ethics*. 2nd edition. New York: Bartlett and Jones, 1994.
5. Walters L, Kahn TJ, eds. *Bibliography of Bioethics*. Washington, DC: Georgetown University. Published annually. On-line as BIOETHICSLINE, National Library of Medicine MEDLARS.

| MEDICAL INDICATIONS | PATIENT PREFERENCES |
|---|---|
| 1. What is patient's medical problem? history? diagnosis? prognosis? <br> 2. Is problem acute? chronic? critical? emergent? reversible? <br> 3. What are goals of treatment? <br> 4. What are probabilities of success? <br> 5. What are plans in case of therapeutic failure? <br> 6. In sum, how can this patient be benefited by medical and nursing care, and how can harm be avoided? | 1. What has the patient expressed about preferences for treatment? <br> 2. Has patient been informed of benefits and risks, understood, and given consent? <br> 3. Is patient mentally capable and legally competent? What is evidence of incapacity? <br> 4. Has patient expressed prior preferences, e.g., Advance Directives? <br> 5. If incapacitated, who is appropriate surrogate? Is surrogate using appropriate standards? <br> 6. Is patient unwilling or unable to cooperate with medical treatment? If so, why? <br> 7. In sum, is patient's right to choose being respected to extent possible in ethics and law? |
| QUALITY OF LIFE | CONTEXTUAL FEATURES |
| 1. What are the prospects, with or without treatment, for a return to patient's normal life? <br> 2. Are there biases that might prejudice provider's evaluation of patient's quality of life? <br> 3. What physical, mental, and social deficits is patient likely to experience if treatment succeeds? <br> 4. Is patient's present or future condition such that continued life might be judged undesirable by them? <br> 5. Any plan and rationale to forgo treatment? <br> 6. What plans for comfort and palliative care? | 1. Are there family issues that might influence treatment decisions? <br> 2. Are there provider (physicians and nurses) issues that might influence treatment decisions? <br> 3. Are there financial and economic factors? <br> 4. Are there religious, cultural factors? <br> 5. Is there any justification to breach confidentiality? <br> 6. Are there problems of allocation of resources? <br> 7. What are legal implications of treatment decisions? <br> 8. Is clinical research or teaching involved? <br> 9. Any provider or institutional conflict of interest? |

# CHAPTER 1

# Indications for Medical Intervention

**1.0** This chapter treats the first topic relevant to any ethical problem in clinical medicine, namely, the indications for medical intervention. These indications are the facts about the patient's physical state that suggest the presence of disease and prompt the diagnostic and therapeutic activities that make up modern medical care. They imply the overall goals of medicine: prevention, cure, and care of illness and injury. In most cases, treatment decisions based on medical indications are straightforward and present no obvious ethical problems. For example, a patient complains of frequent urination accompanied by a burning sensation; the physician suspects a urinary tract infection, obtains a confirmatory culture, and prescribes an antibiotic. The physician explains to the patient the nature of the condition and the purpose and action of the medication. The patient obtains the prescription, takes the medication, and is cured of the infection. This case exemplifies clinical ethics, not because it shows an ethical problem, but because the ethics have gone as smoothly as the medicine. Medical indications are clear enough for the physician to make a diagnosis and prescribe an effective therapy to benefit the patient. The patient's preferences coincide with the physician's recommendations, and the patient's quality of life, presently rendered unpleasant by the infection, is improved. Insurance pays the bill, medications are available, and no other complications arise. The ethical principles of respect for autonomy, beneficence and nonmaleficence, justice, and loyalty are satisfied.

In some cases, however, the ethical aspects become ethical problems. Even in the simple case mentioned above, ethical problems would appear if the patient stated that he did not believe in antibiotics, or if the urinary tract infection developed in the last days of a terminal illness, or if the infection was clearly associated with a sexually transmitted disease where sexual partners might be endangered, or if the patient could not pay for the care. Sometimes, these problems can be readily resolved; at other times, they become major obstacles in the management of the case. A clear understanding of the patient's medical status—namely, the nature of the disease, its prognosis, the available treatments and, above all, the goals of intervention—is crucial to the understanding of any ethical problem that might arise in the case.

In this chapter, we focus on the ways in which uncertainty or disagreement about the medical facts of the case can contribute to an ethical problem. The topic of medical indications is explained, the ethical principles relevant to medical intervention, namely, beneficence and nonmaleficence, are defined, and three ethical issues that depend heavily on the indications for medical intervention will be discussed: (1) medical futility; (2) the decision not to resuscitate a patient in the event of cardiorespiratory arrest; (3) the determination of death.

Every discussion of an ethical problem in clinical medicine must begin with a statement of the medical facts. This statement should follow the pattern familiar to medical students and physicians when they present a patient for clinical purposes: presenting complaint, history, results of physical examination, laboratory and other diagnostic studies, presumptive diagnosis and prognosis, and current or planned therapies. In the usual clinical presentation, this review of indications for medical intervention leads to the formulation of recommendations for further diagnostic studies, treatment regimens, and the education of the patient. When the clinical presentation includes an ethical problem, this review clarifies the medical aspects that are significant in the case.

**Case.** Mr. Cure, a 24-year-old white male, who is a graduate student, has been brought to the emergency room by a friend. Previously in good health, he is complaining of severe headache and a stiff neck. Physical examination shows a somnolent but arousable patient with a temperature of 39.5°C, pulse of 115 and regular, BP of 105/50, and respiratory rate of 20/min. Examination of the chest reveals rales in the right base and neurological examination is normal except for nuchal rigidity and a positive Brudzinski's sign. Laboratory studies show a white count of 20,000 with a left shift; chest x-ray demonstrates a right lower lobe infiltrate. After obtaining the patient's consent, a spinal fluid examination reveals cloudy fluid with a white count of 2,000; a gram stain of the fluid shows many gram-positive diplococci. A diagnosis of pneumococcal pneumonia and pneumococcal meningitis is reached.

In this case, the medical indications are the physical and physiological findings that reveal a specific disease for which a specific therapy, namely, administration of antibiotics, is appropriate. There is no suggestion yet that this case poses any ethical problem. However, in Chapter 2, we shall encounter a major ethical problem with Mr. Cure: he will refuse therapy. That refusal will provoke dismay among the physicians and nurses caring for him and will be designated as an ethical problem. In any discussion of this ethical problem, even though the refusal of treatment will be the center of attention, the formal review of the case must begin with a clear exposition of the medical indications. In other words, the analysis should begin, not with the question, "Does a patient have the right to refuse treatment of a life-threatening condition?" but with answers to the question, "What are the medical indications for treatment?"

## 1.1          THE GOALS AND BENEFITS OF MEDICINE

**Beneficence and Nonmaleficence.**  Medicine aims to prevent or cure disease, to treat patients' symptoms, and to improve or maintain their functional abilities. The two ethical principles that are particularly important guides in the attempt to achieve these aims are beneficence and nonmaleficence. The presence of medical indications raises the question, "How can a medical intervention help this patient?" This question reflects one of the central ethical maxims of medical practice, stated in the Hippocratic oath, "I will use treatment to help the sick according to my ability and judgment but never with a view to injury and wrongdoing." Another Hippocratic writing states, "As to diseases make a habit of two things: to help or at least to do no harm" (*Epidemics* I, xi). These maxims reflect the ethical principles of "beneficence," the duty to assist persons in need, and its converse, "nonmaleficence," the duty to refrain from causing harm. These principles are treated extensively in the texts on the philosophical foundations of medical ethics. The ethical responsibilities of physicians are closely tied to their ability to fulfill the goals of medicine in conjunction with the patients' preferences about the goals of their lives. The physician does so by making clinical judgments about diagnosis, therapy, and education based upon the indications presented by the patient. The principles of beneficence and nonmaleficence require the physician to evaluate the potential benefits of any proposed intervention in relation to its risks, make a recommendation to the patient, and solicit the patient's preferences about whether to undergo the treatment. [EB: "Beneficence," I, 243–247; PBE: ch.5, 259–325; ME: ch.2, 29–55; Pellegrino ED, Thomasma D. *For the Patient's Benefit: The Restoration of Beneficence in Health Care.* New York: Oxford University Press, 1988.]

The physician's central responsibility is to use medical expertise to respond to the patient's need for help. That need is usually expressed by a patient's request to learn the significance of physical signs and symptoms that disturb well-being, to have those disturbing signs and symptoms relieved and the underlying disorder cured. The physician benefits the patient by interpreting the patient's presenting complaint in light of the signs and symptoms, the patient's history, the relevant laboratory data and other studies. The physician then makes a diagnosis and recommends a course of action. That course of action will have some or all of the following goals:

1. Promotion of health and prevention of disease
2. Relief of symptoms, pain, and suffering
3. Cure of disease
4. Preventing untimely death
5. Improvement of functional status or maintenance of compromised status
6. Education and counseling of patients regarding their condition and its prognosis
7. Avoiding harm to the patient in the course of care

The achievement of these goals is the benefit of medicine. Frequently, all or most of these goals can be achieved simultaneously. In Mr. Cure's case, the administration of antibiotics should relieve symptoms and cure the disease, thereby preventing Mr.

Cure's death and restoring his health. In addition, Mr. Cure might be immunized with pneumococcal vaccine at the time of discharge, thus achieving the goal of health promotion. Sometimes it is difficult to accomplish all desirable goals for several reasons: (a) uncertainty about the nature of the problem or about the proper course of action, (b) conflict between diverse goals, (c) the difficulty of attaining a positive goal without doing harm. Often the ethical problem in a particular case will arise from lack of clarity about the goals of intervention or from the apparent incompatibility between goals.

*EXAMPLES:*    (a) Chronic fatigue syndrome, a debilitating condition that involves persistent physical exhaustion, joint pain, and psychological depression, may be precipitated by viral infection or may be psychogenic. No antiviral therapy has been effective, and psychiatric intervention does not appear helpful. Both the nature of the problem and the proper course of action are uncertain. Only the goals of education and counseling of the patient are within reach.

(b) A college basketball player is noted to have a life-threatening cardiac arrhythmia and is treated with a beta blocker. This drug suppresses the arrhythmia but decreases the player's exercise capacity and effectiveness in playing basketball. In this case, a trade-off must be made between trying to prolong life by preventing a fatal arrhythmia and compromising functional capacity, i.e., his ability to play well.

(c) Combined antiretroviral therapy (including protease inhibitors) clearly delays the progression of HIV infection, often improves quality of life and prolongs survival. The degree of long-term benefit remains uncertain. These drugs may have certain side effects, particularly nausea, diarrhea, and kidney stones. They require patients to take up to 14 tablets per day in accord with a rigorous schedule and cost approximately $12,000 per year. The use of combination therapy for preventive purposes poses a difficult trade-off between risks and benefits. The goal of delaying symptoms may be compromised by the goal of avoiding harm: in this case, the serious side effects, the burden of the drug regimen, the cost of the drugs, and the uncertain long-term benefits of such a regimen.

**Clinical Judgment.**    When goals of intervention are unclear, or when previously clear goals become cloudy, ethical questions are asked, such as "What are we accomplishing?" "Is the expected outcome worth the effort?" "Do the benefits justify the risks?" Ethical reflection must begin with a realistic evaluation of the goals of intervention. The results of this evaluation must inform the physician's opinion about the possible courses of action and must be presented to the patient or the patient's surrogate. The process by which a physician reaches a clinical judgment requires the ability to gather data, to discern relevant differences, to discard extraneous facts, to reason probabilistically about the possible courses of action, and to recommend the course that seems best.

**Clinical Uncertainty.**    Clinical medicine was described by Osler as "a science of uncertainty and an art of probability." The central task of clinicians is to reduce uncertainty by using data-gathering skills, medical knowledge, and clinical reasoning to reach a diagnosis and propose a plan of care that will best meet the patient's needs. The physician's recommendation can be considered "best," not in some absolute sense, but because, given the available facts and their interpretation, judicious reflection suggests that it responds to the patient's medical needs and meets the patient's overall goals more adequately than other options. In the recent past, the process by which discerning clinicians, faced with clinical uncertainty, attempted to make consistently good decisions was referred to as "clinical judgment." In conjunction with the personal side of medicine—empathy, respect for persons, effective communication skills, and commitment to the patient's interests—clinical judgment constituted the "art of medicine." Physicians know that scientific understanding is often incomplete. They recognize that data gathering and interpreting take place in a complex context of scientific and personal assumptions, and that clinical recommendations often reflect the individual physician's attitudes about risk-avoidance, enthusiasm for intervention, and other personal and professional values. Above all, physicians are aware that each patient is unique and that the presentation of even common conditions can be peculiar. Yet, despite these uncertainties and influences, physicians have believed that clinical judgment was an "art," in which knowledge could be brought to bear on a patient's problem and that the art was, in the last analysis, an intuitive process too complex to be subjected to analysis or scientific study.

In recent years, that traditional view has been challenged. It has been asserted that clinical medicine is a science and that the disciplines of clinical biostatistics, clinical epidemiology, and decision analysis can be utilized to evaluate the quality of both physicians' decisions and patients' outcomes. Scholars began to study the microlevel of bedside clinical decisions and the macrolevel of the quality of health services. These studies revealed that different clinicians in different locales made very different medical judgments about the same sort of problem. Scholars also suggested principles for the reduction of uncertainty: clinical decisions should be based on solid evidence derived from well-conducted, randomized, controlled trials or cohort studies and, absent such evidence, on the less convincing evidence from case controlled studies and expert clinical opinion. That evidence must show that a treatment is effective, that its prospective benefits outweigh harms, and that it represents a good use of limited resources. "Practice guidelines," which guide a physician's reasoning through particular clinical problems, are being developed on the basis of such evidence. The "uncertainty" and "probability" of which Osler spoke remain, but clinical science aims to focus these down into an evidence-based medicine.

The most fundamental change in the relationship between clinical judgment and medical uncertainty has been a gradual shift, over the past few decades, in decisional authority from the physician to the patient. Even advocates of evidence-based medicine conclude that the patient is the best decision-maker because only the patient can assess the goals of treatment, its risks and benefits and the costs of treatment, in the face of clinical uncertainty that will always be present in medicine. One of those advocates has written, "It is the job of the evaluative sciences to conduct technology assessment and outcomes research to estimate the probability for outcomes that matter to patients and to elucidate the importance of patient preferences in choosing treatment." [Wennberg, JE. Social and economic issues in medicine. *Cecil Textbook of Medicine,* 20th ed. Philadelphia: Saunders, 1996, p. 10.]

Physicians also recognize that judgments about medical indications are not wholly derived from facts. Their judgments are colored by personal values in many respects: an activist or conservative attitude about intervention, peer esteem and career advancement, a compassionate or skeptical view of the human condition. Emotions that a physician may be loath to admit may bias outwardly "objective" judgments: anxiety regarding death and disability, dislike of certain sorts of persons or life-styles, racial prejudice, gender bias, repugnance for the aged or retarded, or desire for economic profit. It is important to be aware of the affective aspects of ostensibly objective medical judgments. Clinical judgments are made in a matrix of facts and values susceptible to the influence of negative attitudes that may distort the clinical picture. Sensitivity to positive attitudes, such as empathy, concern or respect, can facilitate communication and enhance clinical judgment. In this chapter, we will consider the clinician's reasoning, based on knowledge, scientific evidence, and the particular data about a patient, that leads to the formulation of a clinical judgment. In the next chapter, we will discuss the role of the patient's preferences in clinical judgment.

**Important Distinctions.**   In order to understand the clinical situation of the patient, certain distinctions that arise from the nature of disease, treatment, and clinical outcome must be appreciated. The ethical aspects of the case will often depend on these distinctions.

   *THE DISEASE:*   Disease conditions may be
   (a) *acute* (having rapid onset, severe symptoms and short course) or *chronic* (with persistent, usually progressive course over a long period),
   (b) *critical* or *emergent* (causing immediate, serious and irreversible functional disabilities, including death, unless treatment is immediately applied) or *noncritical* or *nonemergent* (slowly progressive, even when serious, but not immediately life-threatening),
   (c) *reversible* (course can be altered by definitive, effective therapy) or *irreversible* (symptoms or acute crises can be managed but course progresses inevitably toward death).

   *THE TREATMENT:*   Modalities of intervention may be
   (a) *curative* (a single treatment, such as a course of antibiotics for simple infection or surgical operation for hernia, will definitively correct the disease condition) or *supportive* (relieving symptoms or reducing deterioration over the entire course of a chronic, irreversible disease, such as diabetes),
   (b) *burdensome* (causing adverse effects that are painful, disfiguring or disabling, such as some cancer chemotherapy) or *nonburdensome* (unlikely to have perceptible or serious side

effects, such as moderate exercise for prevention of mild obesity, or antibiotic treatment of acute bladder infection).

The goals of intervention differ in relation to these distinctions. One common ethical problem occurs when a person with a chronic, nonemergent, irreversible disease (such as multiple sclerosis) presents with an acute, emergent and reversible problem (such as a myocardial infarction). The goals of intervention relative to the latter condition must be evaluated in light of the goals proper to the former. For example, a definitive treatment, such as a successful cardiopulmonary resuscitation in a terminally ill cancer patient, may do nothing more than prolong a painful dying. Returning to the case of Mr. Cure, the patient with meningitis (1.0), the goals of medical intervention seem obvious. The patient has pneumococcal meningitis, an acute, critical and reversible medical problem that can be treated easily with a course of antibiotics. We should note, however, that, given certain changes in the medical facts of the case, the goals of intervention would not be so clear. For example, if Mr. Cure were known to be terminally ill due to metastatic cancer or was suffering from an untreatable brain tumor, the goal of reversing an acute, lethal condition would be less obvious.

## 1.1 P   Pediatrics

The description and resolution of ethical problems in pediatrics proceed in the same fashion as in adult medicine. First, the medical indications for diagnostic and therapeutic interventions based upon the patient's physical condition should be reviewed. These indications must reflect the goals of medical practice and the responsibilities of pediatricians.

**Responsibilities and Goals.**   In general, the responsibilities of pediatricians are the same as those of other physicians: to benefit the patient and to refrain from harm. The goals of medical intervention are the same, whether the patient is adult or infant: restoration of health, relief of symptoms, restoration of impaired function, saving life, and preventing untimely death. In pediatric medicine, the exercise of these responsibilities has some special features:

(a) Infants at the beginning of life have no preferences; children are often too immature to formulate preferences.

(b) Parents or guardians have the moral and legal responsibility to act in the child's best interest. If questions arise about conflicts of interest or the wisdom of the parents' or guardians' choices, the scope of their authority may require legal limitation.

(c) The interests of the patient may be affected by the family situation, such as the interest of siblings, economic factors, or religious beliefs. Family values, not only individual preferences, shape the interpretation of benefits for the child.

(d) As children mature, their preferences become increasingly important in reaching decisions about appropriate treatment.

These features of pediatric medicine may modify the exercise of the basic responsibilities of physicians. In particular, the duty to respect the choices of autonomous persons differs significantly when the person with whom the physician communicates is a parent or a guardian rather than a patient who is incapable of autonomous choice. Practitioners in pediatric specialties may be held to a more stringent duty to formulate an independent judgment of what course would be in the patient's best interest and to test and even challenge proxy decisions against this standard.

## 1.2          DECISIONS TO FORGO INEFFICACIOUS
##              OR FUTILE INTERVENTIONS

A patient may be so seriously ill or injured that sound clinical judgment would suggest that the goals of restoration of health and function are unattainable and, thus, certain medical interventions are not indicated or should be limited. These cases present themselves in several ways: the moribund patient, the terminal patient, and the "hopelessly ill" patient. A single case, that of Mrs. Care, with some clinical variations, can illustrate these three situations.

**Case.**   Mrs. Care, a 48-year-old married woman with two children, was diagnosed as having multiple sclerosis (MS) 15 years ago. Her initial symptoms consisted of numbness and weakness of her right leg and decreased visual acuity in the left eye. These signs resolved, but two years later she developed spasticity and weakness in her left leg. During the past 12 years, the patient has experienced progressive deterioration. She developed severe spasticity in both legs, requiring canes, then a walker, and finally full use of a wheelchair. She is now blind in one eye, with markedly decreased vision in the other. When Betaseron became available, she received a one-year trial of the new medication but failed to show a response. Since developing an atonic bladder five years ago, she has required an indwelling Foley catheter and has developed several urinary tract infections. She has several times been to the hospital for management of pyelonephritis and urosepsis. She has difficulty controlling oral secretions and has been hospitalized twice in the last year for aspiration pneumonia. In the course of the last year, she has become profoundly depressed, uncommunicative even with close family and refuses to rise from bed. During the entire course of her illness, she has refused to discuss the issue of terminal care, saying she found such discussion depressing and discouraging.

### 1.2.1  The Moribund Patient

"Moribund" literally means "about to die." Certain clinical conditions indicate with clarity that the patient's organ systems are disintegrating rapidly and irreversibly. Death can be expected within hours.

**Case.**   Mrs. Care, in the advanced stages of MS, suffers from deep decubitus ulcers and osteomyelitis, neither of which has responded to treatment efforts, including skin grafts. During the past month, the patient has been admitted three times to the ICU with aspiration pneumonia and has required mechanical ventilation. Four days after her most recent hospital discharge, she is brought to the ER by paramedics. She is noted to be septic, with a BP of 60/40, and arterial pH of 6.92, and to have agonal respirations. Should she be intubated?

*COMMENT:*   In this situation, it can be argued that intubation is not medically indicated. Medical intervention at this point is sometimes called "futile," that is, offering no therapeutic benefit to the patient. In this case, the word "futile" has its most basic meaning, sometimes called "physiological futility," a condition in which it is scientifically impossible to recover despite any medical intervention and from which no patient is ever known to have recovered. The concept of futility is more fully discussed below (1.2.2e).

*RECOMMENDATION:*   Mrs. Care is moribund. Her death will take place within hours. Interventions such as intubation might delay the time of death for a few hours, but will not change the course. None of the goals of medicine can be attained, even preventing an untimely death: death can only briefly be postponed. This is not an independent and overriding goal in the absence of any other. Thus, intubation is not indicated. The physician should strongly recommend that it be withheld. Indeed, some ethicists would take an even stronger position: the physician need not offer intubation as an option when the intervention is physiologically futile.

### 1.2.2  The Terminal Patient

There is no standard clinical definition of "terminal." The word is often loosely used to refer to any patient with a lethal disease. The term should be applied only to those patients who experienced clinicians expect will die from a specified disease, despite appropriate treatment, in a relatively short period of time, measured in days, weeks, or several months at most. It should be noted that, under Medicare and Medicaid eligibility rules, reimbursement for hospice care requires a diagnosis of a terminal condition with a prognosis of six months or less to live. This is an administrative rather than a clinical definition of terminal. We believe that a diagnosis of terminal condition, in contrast to a life-threatening condition, should be made cautiously. It is perilous to predict precisely how long a terminal patient will live. More than a few studies have shown that even experienced clinicians are notoriously inaccurate in such predictions.

**Case.**  Mrs. Care is living at home. She requires assistance in all activities of daily life and is confined to bed. She has become quite confused and disoriented. She begins to experience breathing difficulties. She is brought to the emergency department. She is now unresponsive, has a high fever and labored respirations. Chest x-ray reveals diffuse haziness suggestive of adult respiratory distress syndrome; arterial blood gases show a $P_{O_2}$ of 35, $P_{CO_2}$ of 85, and pH of 7.02. Cardiac studies demonstrate an acute anteroseptal myocardial infarction. Neurological and pulmonary consultants agree that she has primary neuromuscular respiratory insufficiency. Should Mrs. Care be admitted to the intensive care unit and intubated?

*COMMENT:*  This acute episode is clearly life-threatening. Various interventions might delay Mrs. Care's demise. A respirator may improve gas exchange and support perfusion of organ systems; fibrinolytic therapy might limit the evolving infarct. These interventions aim at two of the goals of medicine, support of compromised function and prolongation of life. However, the physician's doubts about efficacy are more fundamental. Given the presence of progressive and irreversible disease in its final stages and radical damage to multiple organ systems, none of medicine's other important goals can be achieved. The patient will certainly never be restored to health; pain and symptoms will not be alleviated; compromised functions will not be restored, but at best substituted for temporarily by mechanical means. The following reflections are relevant:

(a) Considering the complexities of this patient's situation, the probabilities of her recovery to health, or even to her limited condition prior to this hospitalization, approach zero. It can be said with great assurance, based on the experience of clinicians, that she has no chance of improvement. While her pneumonia might be successfully treated, the neuromuscular etiology of the pneumonia, arising from her MS, cannot be reversed. Mrs. Care has entered the terminal phase of her illness and her death is imminent, even though she is not yet moribund. Her survival, even under the best of circumstances, will probably be no more than several weeks. Thus, medical interventions will not effect any improvement, except, perhaps, a temporary relief of pneumonia, and will not promote any of the goals of medicine, with the possible exception of brief prolongation of life in its terminal stage.

(b) From the viewpoint of medical indications, physicians have no obligation to prolong life independent of their obligation to fulfill at least some of the other goals of medicine. The tradition of medical ethics has taken this position. In the Hippocratic writing entitled *The Art*, the physician is advised to "assuage the suffering of the sick, lessen the violence of their diseases and refuse to treat those who are overmastered by their diseases, recognizing that in such cases medicine is powerless." This wise advice prevailed until recently and we believe it should still be honored. Regrettably, contemporary practice too often pursues a prolongation of organic life that, in the absence of any other human capacities, provides no benefit to the patient. This is a failure to recognize, or a refusal to admit, that in such cases medicine can only postpone, not prevent, death.

(c) Objective information that provides prognostic criteria may be useful in determining whether a particular type of intervention will be efficacious. Such objective information may include the patient's diagnosis, physiological condition, functional status, and comorbidities, together with the patient's estimated likelihood of recovery. One approach to developing this data for patients admitted to the ICU is the Acute Physiological and Chronic Health Evaluation (APACHE). This system combines an acute physiological score, the Glasgow coma score, age, and a chronic disease score to estimate a patient's risk of dying during an ICU admission. Such an analysis done for this patient with pneumonia, ARDS, and acute myocardial infarction would show that the probability of her surviving this ICU admission is extremely low. Even though probability is not equivalent to certainty, it is here, as everywhere else in medicine, a sound basis for clinical judgment. [Knaus WA, Wagner DP, Draper EA, et al. APACHE III Prognostic System. Risk prediction of hospital mortality for critically ill hospitalized adults. *Chest* 1991; 100:1619–1636.]

(d) Mrs. Care has expressed no preferences about the course of her care, and nothing is known from other sources about her preferences. Thus, personal preferences, usually so important in these decisions, are not relevant. The objective data about survival and sound clinical discretion about the probabilities of improvement are determinative in the recommendation to forgo further treatment.

(e) Medical intervention in this case might be called "futile," that is, highly unlikely to produce its desired effect. In 1.2.1 we have seen the term "futility" used to mean "true physiological futility." However, in medicine, where most judgments are probabilistic, futility might be understood as an effort to provide a benefit to a patient that reason and experience suggest is highly likely to fail and whose rare exceptions cannot be systematically produced. The futility concept is often invoked to reach a decision to limit the treatment a patient receives. Physicians sometimes improperly use futility assertions to override a patient's or surrogate's request for a particular medical intervention. The term "futility" has recently been a topic of controversy in medical ethics. Two major questions are debated: First, what level of statistical or experiential evidence is required to assert futility? Second, should physicians ever make decisions on the basis of futility apart from the patient's evaluation of what results should count as futile? The first question pertains to this chapter, the second to Chapter 2. [Schneiderman LJ, Jecker NS, Jonsen AR. Medical futility: response to critiques. *Ann Intern Med* 1996; 125:669–674; Medical Futility: Demands, Duties, Dilemmas. Special Section. *Cambridge Quarterly of Healthcare Ethics* 1993; 2 (2).]

The quantitative aspect of clinical futility requires a probabilistic judgment that an intervention is highly unlikely to produce the desired result. This judgment arises from general clinical experience and, occasionally, from clinical studies that demonstrate very low rates of success for particular interventions (it has been suggested that if soundly designed clinical studies reveal less than 1 percent chance of success, an intervention should be considered futile).

*EXAMPLE:*   A study of 865 patients who required mechanical ventilation after bone marrow transplantation showed no survivors among the 383 patients who had lung injury, hepatic or renal failure and required more than four hours of ventilator support. Such a study suggests that it would be futile to intubate patients with these conditions or to continue ventilation after four hours. [Rubenfeld GD, Crawford SW: Withdrawing life support for medically ventilated recipients of bone marrow transplantation: a case for evidence-based qualitative guidelines. *Ann Intern Med* 1996; 125:625–633.]

(f) Despite debates about the meaning of futility, the concept is useful in medical ethics. First, it introduces a note of realism into excessive medical optimism. Second, it provides the opportunity to open an honest discussion with patients and families about appropriate care. Third, it calls for a careful investigation of the literature about the efficacy of proposed treatments in particular situations. Fourth, it allows consideration of care to focus on what realistically can be done for the patient under the circumstances and to make a case for nontreatment. It is important to note that physicians should never use futility, except in its most basic sense of physiological futility, to justify unilateral decision-making, nor to avoid a difficult conversation with patient or family. Futility should never be invoked when the real problem is frustration with a difficult case or to reflect the physician's negative evaluation of the patient's future quality of life (chapter 3). Finally, a futility claim by itself does not justify rules or guidelines devised by third-party payers to avoid paying for care (Chapter 4).

(g) In many cases, several reasons converge to justify the recommendation that life-sustaining interventions be forgone: medical intervention becomes increasingly futile, patients may have indicated in some way that they do not wish their life sustained (Chapter 2), and continued life will be of poor quality (Chapter 3). Although this convergence of reasons is usually persuasive to physicians and to surrogates, it may happen that one or another

of the reasons is unclear or that the parties interpret them differently. Should surrogates disagree with a recommendation to
forgo treatment, it is often easier for physicians to capitulate to a
surrogate's demands than to insist that further intervention will
be futile. We believe that the use of life-sustaining interventions
that are not medically beneficial must be justified by the particular circumstances of the case or mandated by specific legal
order. Physicians should not postpone death only to avoid dealing
with the appropriateness of continued medical intervention.

   *RECOMMENDATION:*   A clinical judgment that medical intervention is futile, that is, unlikely to achieve any of the goals of
medical treatment or, if it does so, will achieve them in a minimal or transitory way, provides a sound basis for recommending
that interventions be forgone. Thus, admission of Mrs. Care to
the intensive care unit for treatment of pneumonia, ARDS, myocardial infarction, and respiratory failure is not ethically obligatory. The objective data, linked with clinical experience, provide
reasonable grounds for forgoing further treatment. Everything
that ought to be done has been done (note that "ought to be
done" refers to those actions that fulfill ethical obligations, not to
everything technically possible). This should be communicated
to the family with the recommendation that Mrs. Care be treated
in a quiet room and receive only those measures to keep her
comfortable. No further tests should be done. Should patient or
family request treatment judged inefficacious by physicians, an
ethical problem appears: this sort of conflict will be discussed in
Chapter 2 and Chapter 4.

### 1.2.3   Patients with Progressive, Lethal Disease

Certain diseases follow a course of slow and sometimes occult destruction of the body's physiological processes. Patients who suffer
such diseases may experience their effects continually or inter-
mittently and with varying severity. Eventually, the disease itself
or some associated pathology will cause their death. Mrs. Care illustrates the features of this condition. Multiple sclerosis cannot be
cured; progressive neurological complications that include spasticity, loss of mobility, neurogenic bladder, respiratory insufficiency,
and occasionally dementia are also incurable. Still, some interventions, such as treatment of infection, can relieve symptoms, maintain some level of function, and prolong life.

**Case.** For the first decade after her diagnosis with MS, Mrs. Care maintained high spirits. While she did not like to discuss her disease or its prognosis, she seemed to understand the progressive and lethal nature of her condition. However, in the last few years, she has begun to speak frequently of "getting this over," and has become deeply depressed. She has accepted several trials of antidepressant medications, but these did not improve her mental condition. As serious urinary tract and respiratory infections became more frequent, she grudgingly submitted to treatment.

*COMMENT:* Patients in this condition are not "terminal" even though the disease from which they suffer is incurable. However, they may from time to time experience acute, critical episodes which, if not treated, would lead to their death. If successfully treated, the patient will be restored to their "baseline." In a sense, they are, at each episode, "potentially terminal." A discouraged patient may consider any intervention to be futile. It may occur to such patients and to their physicians that these episodes offer an opportunity to end their progressive decline. Recall the old medical maxim, "Pneumonia is the old person's friend." In such a situation, the issues require a careful review of medical indications, since the patient's prognosis, with or without treatment, must be clearly understood. However, the more salient questions concern patient preferences and quality of life. Thus, the ethical dimensions of such cases will be discussed in Chapters 2 and 3.

## 1.2.4 P  Decisions to Forgo Inefficacious or Futile Interventions for Children

With infants and children, as with adults, recommendations must sometimes be made about the appropriate forms of care when death appears imminent. Although it is often psychologically and emotionally more difficult to accept the death of an infant or child, pediatricians must sometimes recommend that certain interventions are not medically indicated because they are futile, providing no or only minimal benefits, or because they impose burdens disproportionate to their benefits.

**Case I.** An anencephalic infant is born to a mother who had no prenatal care. Large portions of the cranium are absent and the forebrain and much of the brainstem are missing. The infant is gasping at birth.

**Case II.**   A fetus is delivered by spontaneous abortion at 23 weeks gestation, weighing 410 g and is asphyxiated at birth.

**Case III.**   Jason, a 4-year-old boy, absent from home for about two hours, is found at the bottom of a nearby pond. When drawn from the water, he is limp, with grayish pallor, and cold. His father initiates mouth-to-mouth resuscitation with no response. The emergency service arrives eight minutes later. Resuscitative efforts stimulate a few irregular heartbeats but no stable rhythm after ten minutes.

**Case IV.**   Kerry was born at 23 weeks gestation weighing 590 grams. In the delivery room, she required intubation and ventilation; Apgar scores were 2 at one minute and 5 at five minutes. Kerry had severe hyaline membrane disease and was started on surfactant replacement. Initially in 80 percent oxygen with high-pressure ventilator settings, Kerry was weaned down to 30 percent oxygen. Kerry's anterior fontanel was noted to be tense, and a head ultrasound revealed a bilateral grade IV intracerebral hemorrhage with associated periventricular leukomalacia. On the fifth day of life, Kerry had surgery for removal of all but 20 cm of necrotic terminal ileum. The infant then develops *Candida* sepsis.

**Case V.**   Amy was diagnosed with acute myelogenous leukemia (AML) at age 8. She received a course of chemotherapy, resulting in a remission after six months. Three months later she relapsed. An allogeneic bone marrow transplantation was performed with her 17-year-old sister as a compatible donor. Again, after several months, Amy's cancer returned. Her parents requested more chemotherapy, which her oncologist advised would be very unlikely to succeed. Despite a course of experimental chemotherapy, Amy's disease progressed. After two difficult months, Amy, who had been a cheerful patient, became very discouraged and depressed. Her parents and her sister urged her to continue the treatment. Amy, now 10 years old, asks why she "has to keep doing this?"

*COMMENT:*   Reasonable clinical judgments of futility or inefficacy are a sound justification for a decision not to intervene or to discontinue medical interventions. In such cases, physicians should recommend that nonbeneficial treatments be withheld or withdrawn. Futility claims should never be used as a callous substitute for empathy with parents whose children are dying. [Jecker

NS, Pagon RA, Fost NC. Futile treatment. In: Goldworth A, et al. *Ethics and Perinatology.* New York: Oxford University Press, 1995.]

*RECOMMENDATIONS:* In all the above cases, it is reasonable to judge that interventions to sustain organic functions will be incapable of restoring these functions to independent activity. In Case I, futility consists in the total inability to correct the cranial and cerebral lesion and in the evidence drawn from experience that none of these babies survive more than a few days. In Case II, no infant of that birthweight and gestational age is known to have survived under current medical regimens. In Case III, resuscitative efforts can be discontinued. There is no reasonable possibility that any further efforts will restore normal cardiac rhythms. In Case IV, lung disease has improved somewhat with surfactin and may continue to improve, even to the point of discontinuing respiratory support. Neurological function and alimentary tract are badly damaged. The probability of surviving *Candida* infection is extremely remote. In Case V, further treatment has only the most remote probability of attaining remission and none of cure; in addition, Amy's emotional response to the prospect of further treatment should be respected, as discussed in Chapter 2. It is ethically correct to recommend withholding or withdrawing interventions in all cases. Should parents refuse this recommendation, the comments at 2.7.5 P are relevant.

**Case VI.**  Patrick was born at 35 weeks gestation after his mother went into premature labor precipitated by polyhydramnios. A prenatal ultrasound, done at 22 weeks gestation, demonstrated a left-sided diaphragmatic hernia. Vigorous at birth, Patrick was immediately intubated and ventilated due to the rapid onset of cyanosis and respiratory distress. In spite of high pressures on the ventilator and 100 percent oxygen, Patrick's arterial oxygen never went above 60 torr nor did his carbon dioxide go below 50 torr. Inhaled nitric oxide and high-frequency ventilation failed to improve oxygenation and ventilation. Chest radiograph showed that Patrick had a large hernia with stomach, intestine, and liver located in his left thorax. His right lung also appeared hypoplastic. The neonatologists considered extracorporeal membrane oxygenation (ECMO).

*COMMENT:*  ECMO is used as therapy for severe pulmonary hypertension. It is a procedure whereby blood is diverted out of the body and the infant's oxygenation and ventilation are supported while vessels of the lungs progressively relax. ECMO has improved the survival of infants with pulmonary hypertension. However, with diaphragmatic hernia, both lungs are underdeveloped and thus may not support normal oxygenation and ventilation even with ECMO. While there are currently no certain predictors that discriminate between those who will benefit from ECMO and those who will not, prematurity, gestational age at diagnosis, and extent of lung hypoplasia seem significant. In Patrick's case, a judgment of futility is not unreasonable, although it is always difficult to refrain from a potentially life-saving technology in the face of certain death.

**Case VII.**   At 24 weeks gestation, a fetus was diagnosed by ultrasound as having severe diaphragmatic hernia: most of the abdominal viscera were herniated into the left chest, and there was almost no visible lung.

*COMMENT:*   Diaphragmatic hernia of this severity is thought to be incompatible with postnatal life. The parents of this fetus have four options: (a) terminate the pregnancy, (b) no supportive care after birth, allowing early death, (c) aggressive postnatal care, including respiratory support, ECMO, and surgical correction, (d) immediate fetal surgical repair. Postnatal care will be in all likelihood futile, since the child will have almost no lung to support respiratory function. Fetal surgical repair is theoretically the most efficacious approach, but is experimental and should be chosen only in light of the criteria for clinical research, discussed in Chapter 4.

*RECOMMENDATION:*   The recommendation of physicians to these parents should stress that any intervention is likely to be inefficacious and that the more aggressive postnatal interventions are likely to be more burdensome than beneficial to the infant.

## 1.3                     ORDERS NOT TO RESUSCITATE

One form of medical intervention, cardiopulmonary resuscitation (CPR), deserves careful attention under the topic of indications for medical intervention. Cardiopulmonary resuscitation consists of a set of techniques designed to restore circulation and respiration in the event of acute cardiac or cardiopulmonary arrest. CPR, in its simplest form of mouth-to-mouth insufflation and chest compression, is taught to lay persons for use in emergency situations. In hospitals, advanced CPR is usually carried out by a trained team who respond to an urgent call. Advanced CPR techniques include closed-chest compression, intubation with assisted ventilation, electroconversion of defibrillation, cardiotonic and vasopressive drugs, and intubation for support of ventilation.

The Joint Commission of Health Care Organizations requires that hospitals have a formal policy regarding CPR. Usually, policy will require that CPR be a standing order, that is, it is to be carried out without a specific order on any patient who suffers a cardiac or respiratory arrest. Only when a specific order is issued that CPR is not to be done may it be omitted. This order is called Do Not Attempt Resuscitation (DNAR) or denoted by various circumlocutions such as "No Code Order." The omission of CPR after cardiopulmonary arrest will result inevitably in the death of the patient.

The decision about nonresuscitation is a complex one. Three crucial considerations must be assessed: the first is the judgment that CPR would be futile, that is, that the resuscitation would be very unlikely to succeed or, if it did, another arrest would soon follow. The second important aspect of the Order Not to Resuscitate concerns the preferences of the patient, if known, and the third pertains to the expected quality of life of the patient for whom resuscitation succeeds. The first aspect, the medical futility of the intervention will be treated here; patient preferences and quality of life will be discussed in Chapters 2 and 3. All three aspects must be assessed in any decision to write a DNAR order.

## 1.3.1   Medical Indications and Contraindications for CPR

All persons who suffer unexpected cardiopulmonary arrest for a known or unknown cause and who are not known to be terminally and irreversibly ill should be resuscitated. This is made clear in the Standards for CPR:

> The purpose of cardiopulmonary resuscitation is the prevention of sudden, unexpected death. Cardiopulmonary resuscitation is not indicated in certain situations, such as in cases of terminal, irreversible illness where death is not unexpected. [Standards and guidelines for cardiopulmonary resuscitation (CPR) and emergency cardiac care (ECC). *JAMA* 1980; 244:453.]

*COMMENT:*   (a) Cardiopulmonary resuscitation is inappropriate medical practice in the case of cardiopulmonary arrest that occurs as the anticipated end of a terminal illness or after maximal efforts to save the patient have failed in the emergency department or ICU. CPR need not be applied to patients who are likely to succumb to their basic disease in a short time or to patients in a persistent vegetative state. For such patients, a DNAR order should be written. The inflexibility of many hospital CPR policies may cause conflict for clinicians in particular cases when DNAR orders have not been written. Ideally, a DNAR policy will permit exceptions to the rule of a written order when CPR is clearly not medically indicated, and it has not yet been possible to enter the order.

(b) DNAR orders are usually first considered when the patient is in a terminal condition and death appears to be imminent. A large multicenter study of DNAR orders written in ICUs showed that fewer than 2 percent of patients who had DNAR orders survived to be discharged from the hospital. Many DNAR policies contain the phrase, "when death is imminent." Increasingly, however, nonterminally ill patients, many of whom have chronic incurable diseases such as metastatic cancer and AIDS, but who are not moribund or acutely terminally ill, discuss DNAR orders with their physicians as a component of advanced care planning. Many of these patients are prepared to die peacefully without resuscitation attempts because they are concerned that even if they are "successfully" resuscitated, they may experience anoxic brain damage or some other functional impairment. For nonterminally ill patients who have DNAR orders, several published studies have shown survival to discharge to be as high as 50 to 70 percent. Studies have shown that the timing of DNAR orders varies among hospitals and that the three best predictors of the timing of DNAR orders (in decreasing frequency) are: patient preferences, poor prognosis measured by less than 50 percent chance of surviving two months, and age greater than 75 (regardless of prognosis). [Support Principal Investigators. A controlled trial to improve care for seriously ill hospitalized patients. *JAMA* 1995; 274:1591–1598.]

(c) Studies also indicate that even in terminally ill patients, DNAR orders are underused (as measured by the number of patients who had indicated a preference for such orders in relation to those for whom orders were actually written) because of a lack of communication and discussion among physicians, patients, and families. In our view, it is the responsibility of physicians to initiate DNAR discussions with decisionally capable patients (or with the surrogates of patients who are decisionally incapacitated) who are terminally ill or have incurable disease with estimated 50 percent survival of less than three years, or who are admitted with acute, life-threatening conditions or who bring up other issues about advanced care planning. [Hakim RB, Teno JM, Harrell FE, et al. Factors associated with Do-Not-Resuscitate orders: patients' preferences, prognosis and physicians' judgments. *Ann Intern Med* 1996; 125:284–293.]

(d) Recent studies have shown that CPR is not effective in restoring cardiac function for certain classes of patients or has only a low probability of doing so. Even when CPR succeeds at the time of the arrest, relatively few of these patients survive to discharge. Studies show a survival-to-discharge rate of about 15 percent, and suggest that survival was more likely in patients with respiratory rather than cardiac arrest, in witnessed cardiac arrests, in patients who had few comorbid conditions, and in patients who experienced a short duration of CPR. In general, studies show that immediate success of in-hospital resuscitation is 30 to 40 percent, but only 15 percent of these survive to discharge. Survival is much less likely in patients with preexisting hypotension, renal failure, sepsis, pneumonia, acute stroke, metastatic cancer, AIDS, or homebound life-style. For the small percentage of patients who survive to discharge, two studies have shown good long-term prognosis, with 33 to 54 percent survivals. Although some studies suggested that age greater than 70 is a negative prognostic feature, other studies have not confirmed this. It is essential that patients, families, and physicians have this kind of information on the benefits and risks of CPR so that they can make informed decisions about using CPR or choosing DNAR status. [Karetzky M, Zubair M, Paraikh J. Cardiopulmonary resuscitation in intensive care unit and non-intensive care unit patients: immediate and long term survival. *Arch Intern Med* 1995; 155:1277–1280; Robinson GR, Hess D. Postdischarge survival and functional status following in-hospital cardiopulmonary resuscitation. *Chest* 1994; 105:991–996; Saklyen M, Liss H, Makert R. In hospital cardiopulmonary resuscitation: survival in one hospital and literature review. *Medicine* (Baltimore) 1995: 74:163–175.]

(e) Ordinarily, the permission of the patient to omit CPR is required, provided that the patient is capable of participating in the decision. However, there is currently debate among medical ethicists about whether it is ever ethically acceptable for a physician to make a decision not to resuscitate without consulting the patient or the patient's surrogate or even in the face of objections from the patient or surrogate. Those in favor of not consulting argue that a medical judgment that CPR would be futile means that it is not indicated, that is, it would not attain the goals of medicine and thus need not be offered as an option to the patient. Those who reject this position argue it violates the standard of informed consent: the patient should always have the right to refuse or choose CPR, because the quality of the patient's surviving life is a judgment that the patient alone should make, and that even the remote chance of successful resuscitation may be of value to the patient. Further, they assert that there is lack of agreement on what probability of survival constitutes futility and that physicians are inconsistent in their application of the futility concept. Finally, unilateral decisions are open to bias against racial minorities and other patients who might be objects of discrimination. If the patient is mentally incapacitated, the family and/or the designated surrogate should be informed. If the physician has concluded that CPR would be futile, all parties should be so informed and a DNAR order, based on that rationale, entered. [Tomlinson T, Brody H. Futility and the ethics of resuscitation. *JAMA* 1990; 318:43; Youngner S. Who defines futility? *JAMA* 1988; 260:2094; Youngner S. Futility in context. *JAMA* 1990; 264:1294; Blackhall LJ. Must we always use CPR? *NEJM* 1987; 317:1281.]

**EXAMPLES.**    (a) Mr. Cure, the young man with severe headache and stiff neck, is admitted to the hospital with a diagnosis of meningitis. He refuses antibiotic therapy. Within a few minutes, he suffers a cardiac arrest. The intern, aware of the patient's refusal of necessary therapy, wonders whether resuscitation should be initiated.

(b) Mrs. Care, the patient with multiple sclerosis, has been admitted to the hospital for treatment of pneumonia and evaluation of her breathing difficulties. Neurological consultation concludes that her respiratory insufficiency is secondary to the advancing muscular and neurological deterioration of MS. Should a DNAR be written?

(c) L.M., a 68-year-old man without family, has been diagnosed with tight aortic stenosis (.3-mm orifice) and scheduled for valve replacement surgery. While in his doctor's office, he suffers a cardiac arrest. No discussion of CPR has taken place. Should he be resuscitated?

**RECOMMENDATIONS:**    Mr. Cure, even though he has refused antibiotic therapy for a life-threatening condition, should certainly be resuscitated. The reason for his refusal has not been adequately elucidated, and the refusal of a particular therapy should not be taken as equivalent to refusal of all therapy. Failure to resuscitate would constitute serious medical negligence and ethical fault. In the case of Mrs. Care, recommendations should be made to the family that even if CPR succeeds, the patient would survive only a short time. If the family concurs, a DNAR order should be entered. If the family disagrees, CPR should be provided in the event of a cardiac arrest. In some cases, demands by family may appear excessive or unreasonable: these situations should be managed in accord with the advice stated in Chapter 4. Mr. L.M. may exemplify "physiological futility." His stenosis is very severe and even vigorous resuscitation is highly unlikely to restore adequate cardiac output. His physician, knowing his condition, might reasonably refrain from resuscitative attempts, which might have nothing but traumatic effects.

## 1.3.2    Documentation of DNAR Order

Attending physicians should clearly write and sign the DNAR in the orders section of the patient's chart. The progress notes should include the medical facts and opinion underlying the order and a summary of the discussion with patient, consultants, staff, and family. The status of the order should be reviewed at regular intervals in view of the condition of the patient and should be changed if the condition of the patient warrants it. Everyone involved with the care of the patient should be informed of the DNAR order and its rationale. Because studies have shown that the term DNAR means different things to different practitioners, the physician writing the order must be careful to document the specific terms of the order. Decisions to withhold or withdraw interventions other than DNAR should be noted by the writing of specific orders rather than relying on the DNAR order to cover a wide range of decisions. The writing of a DNAR order should have no direct bearing on any treatment other than CPR. Physicians should recall that a significant number of patients for whom DNAR orders are written leave the hospital.

Patients for whom DNAR orders have been written in the hospital may be discharged with the expectation that they will die soon. It sometimes happens that these patients suffer a crisis and family members summon emergency services. On arrival, the emergency personnel are required to resuscitate. Some states have enacted legislation to validate a "portable DNAR" which testifies clearly that the patient should not be resuscitated. In the absence of such protection, terminal and moribund patients are sometimes returned to the hospital for undesired and futile treatment. On discharge from the hospital, these patients and their families should be given clear instructions about how to deal with an acute, and potentially terminal, situation.

### 1.3.3   "Partial Codes"

Occasionally, one hears the expression "partial code." This refers to the practice of calling a code but separating the various interventions that constitute resuscitation and using them selectively: thus, chest compression, assisted breathing by AMBU bag and cardiotonic drugs may be ordered, but intubation omitted. We advise that cardiopulmonary resuscitation be defined as an integrated set of procedures that should all be applied in the absence of a DNAR order to reverse all effects of cardiac arrest. Yet physicians and patients may develop a plan for resuscitation that omits intubation: such a plan may be respected if its rationale is made clear. Finally, the infamous "slow code," in which personnel respond slowly and without energy to an arrest, is reprehensible. It merely represents the failure to come to a timely and clear decision about a patient's resuscitation status. It is crass dissimulation.

### 1.3.4   DNAR Orders in the Operating Room

Occasionally patients for whom a DNAR order has been written, for example, patients with terminal cancer, require a palliative surgical procedure such as emergency correction of a bowel obstruction to relieve pain or the elective insertion of a gastrostomy tube or central venous catheter. The question has been raised whether the DNAR order should be suspended automatically during anesthesia or surgery so that the patients would be resuscitated if they experienced a perioperative cardiac arrest. The arguments favoring this policy are that anesthesia and surgery place patients at high risk for cardiac and hemodynamic instability; most arrests in the operating room are reversible due to the skill and equipment instantly available; in consenting to surgery, the patient gives implied consent for resuscitation; surgeons and anesthesiologists should not be prevented from treating the anticipated consequences of their own interventions and they do not wish deaths of terminally ill patients to be considered surgical deaths when standard resuscitative techniques have been prohibited. The majority of anesthesiologists, in one study, assumed DNAR suspension, and only half of these discussed this assumption with the patient or surrogate.

Those opposed to automatic suspension of DNAR orders note that such a policy ignores patients' rights and violates the standards of informed consent. They recommend instead a policy of "required reconsideration." The patient who enters the surgical suite faces a different risk/benefit situation: this merits a new evaluation of the DNAR order. A specific discussion between the attending physicians and surgeons and the patient or surrogates should raise the question; the parties should discuss the relevant considerations and either affirm or suspend the order in anticipation of surgery. The major professional associations of surgeons, anesthesiologists, and nurses have endorsed this policy, and we recommend it as the most prudent course. We also advise that if a competent patient, after reconsideration, wishes a preexisting DNAR order to stand, resuscitation should not be attempted in the event of an intrasurgical arrest. [Truog R. Do Not Resuscitate Orders: during anesthesia and surgery. *Anesthesiology* 1991; 74:606; Clemency MV, Thompson NJ. Do Not Resuscitate Orders and the anesthesiologists: a survey. *Anesth Analg* 1993; 76:395–401; Walker RM. DNAR in the OR: resuscitation as operative risk. *JAMA* 1991; 266: 2407–2412; Statement of the American College of Surgeons. Advanced Directive by Patients: Do Not Resuscitate in the operating room. *Bull Am Coll Surg* 1994; 63:29; Cohen CB, Cohen PJ. Do-not-resuscitate orders in the operating room. *NEJM* 1991; 325:1879–1882.]

### 1.3.5 P  Orders Not to Resuscitate Infants and Children

In general, the conditions for an order not to initiate cardiopulmonary resuscitation are the same for a child as for an adult, with the exception of the patient's consent. However, resuscitation of the asphyxiated newborn raises special questions.

**Case I.**  A baby is delivered by spontaneous abortion at 23 weeks gestation, weighing 410 grams, and is asphyxiated at birth.

**Case II.**  An infant, born at 33 weeks gestation, appears to be microcephalic, with low-set, posteriorly rotated ears. A single umbilical artery is noted, in addition to an oddly shaped chest. The birth had been precipitous, the mother having received Demerol IM 1 hour preceding. Apgar score is 1 at 1 minute; heart rate 80 beats/min.

*COMMENT AND RECOMMENDATION:*    In Case I, it is ethically correct to determine before birth or at birth not to resuscitate. Experience indicates that even if resuscitated, this very small premature infant will not survive. In Case II, resuscitation should be attempted, since the nature of the child's congenital problems is not clear and the depressed state of the infant is possibly due to the presence of narcotics. Resuscitation and evaluation do not rule out a later decision to withdraw treatment, based either on medical indications or on quality of life considerations as discussed in Chapter 3.

## 1.4                    CARE OF THE DYING PATIENT

The decision to terminate specific forms of treatment or not to resuscitate does not imply the termination of care for the patient. It is frequently noted that after a DNAR order is written, attention to the patient's needs diminishes. This is unethical for two reasons: first, since in some series more than 50 percent of patients for whom DNAR orders have been written survive to discharge, these patients require continued appropriate care. Second, it is a failure to recognize that when the goals of curing are exhausted, the goals of caring must be reinforced. Attention to relief of pain and discomfort and enhancement of the patient's ability to interact with family and friends become predominant goals. The medical proverb is pertinent: Cure sometimes, relieve occasionally, comfort always. Particular issues in care of the dying patient, such as pain control, are discussed in Chapter 3. [EB: "Hospice and End of Life Care," II, 1157–1160.]

### 1.4.1    Legal Implications

It is a general principle of the law of medical negligence that expert witnesses testifying that a particular medical intervention is not indicated stands as a defense against a charge of negligence. Thus, if it can be demonstrated that, in view of good medical practice, some intervention would be judged futile, as offering no medical benefit, presumably physicians are safe to recommend that it be omitted. While many judicial decisions have supported the decision to discontinue life-support or to order DNAR, most of these rely on legal interpretations of patients' preferences and on the patient's quality of life, rather than on claims of medical futility alone. We list the most important of these cases in Chapter 3. Two recent cases pertain more directly to futility. In one case (*In re* Wanglie, Minn., 1991) the court supported a surrogate's demand to continue ventilator support for an 87-year-old woman in a persistent vegetative state, although the attending physicians considered it medically inappropriate. In the other (Gilgunn v. MGH, Mass., 1995), a jury trial held the hospital harmless against claims of the family for discontinuing care judged futile by attending physicians whose judgment was endorsed by the hospital's ethics committee. Neither case provides clear guidance for practitioners. We recommend that hospitals formulate policy defining appropriate care and the methods whereby decisions in difficult cases should be made and reviewed. Physicians and hospitals are most justifiably criticized and most likely to get into difficulty when they make unilateral decisions, especially if they have failed to communicate and negotiate with surrogates, consult with colleagues, follow administrative procedures and policies, and seek legal consultation. [Meisel, A. *The Right to Die*. New York: John Wiley and Sons, 1989, Supplement #2, 1992; Miles SH. Informed consent for non-beneficial treatment. *NEJM* 1991;325: 512–515; Capron AM. Abandoning a waning life. *Hastings Center Report* 1995; 25: 24–26.]

**1.4.2 P**  In 1985, the U.S. Congress passed amendments to The Child Abuse Prevention and Treatment and Adoption Reform Act which pertain to clinical decisions about newborns. The regulations based on this legislation are known as "The Baby Doe Rules." These rules are discussed at 4.5.1 P. However, here we note that the rules do not require life-sustaining treatment, "when the provision of such treatment would merely prolong dying, not be effective in ameliorating or correcting all of the infant's life threatening conditions, or otherwise be futile in terms of the survival of the infant." [Child Abuse and Neglect: Prevention and Treatment Program, 50 *Code of Federal Regulations,* April 15, 1985, at 14888.]

One controversial court decision, popularly known as the case of Baby K, is also discussed at 4.5.1 P. That case casts a legal cloud over the futility discussion because it seems to imply that even irreversibly dying infants are entitled to emergency lifesaving care if a parent demands such care. Given the circumstances of the case, the ruling cannot be generalized and clinicians should seek legal counsel about its interpretation. [Annas GJ. Asking the

courts to set the standard of emergency care—the case of Baby
K. *NEJM* 1994; 330:1542–1545.]

**1.5**                        **DETERMINATION OF DEATH**

Medical intervention ceases when the patient is declared dead.
Declaring death is one of the legal duties of physicians. Traditionally, the moment of death was considered to be the time when
a person ceased, and did not resume, communication, movement,
and breathing. The body soon becomes cold and rigid, and putre-
faction sets in. It became customary for physicians to determine
death by noting the absence of respiration and pulse and the fix-
ation of pupils. Thus, the common definition of death, accepted
in medicine and in the law, was "irreversible cessation of circulation and respiration." This is known as the "cardiorespiratory
criterion" of death.

This criterion presupposes loss of the integrating function of
the brainstem. When this function ceases, spontaneous breathing stops, followed by a disintegration of all vital organ systems.
The unoxygenated brain rapidly loses all cognitive and other
regulatory functions; the unoxygenated heart ceases to beat. In
the 1960s it became possible to maintain respiratory functions
by the use of a mechanical ventilator, which can support oxygen
perfusion even in the absence of brainstem function.

The concept of "brain criteria" for death that would comple-
ment or replace "cardiorespiratory criteria" emerged in the 1960s.
The advent of organ transplantation stimulated interest in this
concept, since its application would make possible the preservation of organs after death. In 1968, the Report of the Ad Hoc
Committee of the Harvard Medical School to Examine the Definition of Brain Death, "A Definition of Irreversible Coma," described certain clinical characteristics of a nonfunctioning brain:
unreceptivity and unresponsivity to external stimuli, no move-
ments or breathing, no reflexes, no discernible electrical activity
in the cerebral cortex as shown by electroencephalogram (EEG).
[Report of the Ad Hoc Committee of the Harvard Medical School
to Examine the Definition of Brain Death. A definition of irreversible coma. *NEJM* 1968; 205:337.]

The use of these "brain criteria" for determination of clinical
death was gradually accepted by legal jurisdictions. However,
there was much confusion about their proper application. In
particular, there was confusion between "total brain death" and
"irreversible coma" (now called "persistent vegetative state," see

3.2). This confusion was the source of ethical and legal problems. Thus, in 1981, the President's Commission for the Study of Ethical Problems in Medicine proposed a model legal statute, The Uniform Definition of Death. As of 1987, this statute had been adopted in legislation by 39 states and the District of Columbia, and in an additional 6 states judicial decisions had upheld the brain death standard.

> An individual who has sustained either (1) irreversible cessation of circulatory and respiratory function, or (2) irreversible cessation of all functions of the entire brain, including the brain stem, is dead. A determination of death must be made in accordance with accepted medical standards. [President's Commission on Ethical Problems in Medicine and Biomedical and Behavioral Research. *Defining Death: A Report on the Medical, Legal, and Ethical Issues in Definition of Death.* Washington, DC: Government Printing Office, 1981.]

The accepted medical standards for clinical diagnosis of death by brain criteria are: no voluntary or involuntary movement except spinal reflexes, no brainstem reflexes (e.g., apnea in the presence of elevated arterial $CO_2$ when mechanical ventilation is temporarily halted, fixed and dilated pupils, no reaction to aural irrigation, absent doll's eyes response), and exclusion of toxic or drug etiology that can cause the above signs. Brain blood flow studies are confirmatory, particularly for children. Electroencephalography, which diagnoses only absence of cortical function, is not sufficient to establish total brain death and is frequently omitted in the presence of the above clinical signs.

In sum, no medical goals are attainable for a person who is dead by either cardiorespiratory criteria or brain criteria. Ordinarily, all interventions should be terminated. The physician has the authority to declare the patient dead; permission from the family to declare a patient dead or to discontinue medical interventions is not required ethically or legally. The family should be sensitively informed that their relative has died. Contextual features of a particular case might suggest a continuation of supportive technology, for example, sensitivity to needs of family and friends of the patient, salvage of a viable fetus from a brain-dead pregnant woman, or retrieval of organs for transplant (Chapter 4).

It is particularly important that physicians distinguish the ethical and legal implications of death by brain criteria from the implications of the persistent vegetative state. Lay persons (and some physicians and nurses) use the term "brain death" when they are referring to persistent vegetative state. This is misleading. The ethical and legal implications of persistent vegetative state are discussed in Chapter 3 (3.2).

Certain philosophical problems about the adequacy of the definition of death by brain criteria remain open to debate. These disputes need not concern those responsible for clinical decisions in this matter. At the present time, physicians can rely on the legal, clinical, and ethical determinations mentioned above. Religious doctrines have generally accepted this definition of death. The notable exception is Orthodox Judaism, where many authorities insist on use of the cardiorespiratory criteria for theological reasons. [EB: "Death, Definition and Determination of," Vol. 1, 529–549; ME: Ch. 12, "Death and Dying," 363–394; Veatch RM. *Death, Dying, and the Biological Revolution: Our Last Quest for Responsibility.* New Haven: Yale University Press, 1989; Rosner F. *Modern Medicine and Jewish Ethics.* Hoboken, New Jersey: Ktav Publishing House, Inc., 1986, 241–254; Truog RD. Is it time to abandon brain death? *Hastings Center Report* 1997; 27 (1):29–37.]

**1.5.1 P** The clinical method of determining death by brain criteria may be used for infants and children, but special caution is advised, since it is assumed, although not proven, that the child's brain is more resistant to insults leading to death. Physicians responsible for making this determination in children should be familiar with the special clinical issues. In addition to the general criteria (e.g., coma, apnea, absence of brainstem function demonstrated by nonreactive pupils, absence of eye movement, flaccid tone and no spontaneous movement other than spinal cord reflexes, and a rule-out of hypothermia and hypotension; EEG and cerebral blood flow studies are confirmatory), pediatricians are advised not to apply the criteria to infants younger than 7 days. For infants between 7 days and 2 months old, two examinations and EEGs should be done, 24 hours apart; for children over 1 year, the observation period should extend over 12 hours. Naturally, the greatest sympathy and understanding must be extended to parents whose children have died. It is particularly important to make clear that death by brain criteria is distinct from persistent vegetative condition: the term "brain death" confuses the two and should be avoided. Similarly, pediatricians should not speak of "removing life-support" in situations where ventilators are supporting breathing after a determination of death by brain criteria: such language only reinforces the mistaken notion that the parents have "let their child die." [Task Force on Brain Death in Children. Guidelines for the determination of brain death in children. *Pediatrics* 1987; 80:298–299; Kaufman HH ed. *Pediatric Brain Death and Organ/Tissue Retrieval: Medical, Ethical and Legal Aspects.* New York: Plenum Press, 1989.]

**1.6**                               **SUMMARY**

Chapter 1 treats the first topic that must be considered in defining and analyzing an ethical problem in clinical medicine, indications for medical treatment. These indications consist of an accurate presentation of the patient's complaint, diagnosis, and prognosis with a view toward determining what benefits, that is, what goals of medical care, should be sought for the patient. Ethical questions arise when the goals are not clear or when goals conflict. Medical indications must be clearly formulated by physicians in order that they, their patients, and families of patients can understand the range of medically feasible options in the case. Once the medical options are clarified, the other topics—patient preference, quality of life, and contextual features—will be considered in order. In certain situations, the topic of medical indications is particularly important in formulating the ethical justification for forgoing treatment. When death has been declared, no medical indications exist to continue any interventions. When intervention is judged futile, the ethical obligation to provide it or to offer it as an option is attenuated. In all decisions to forgo life-sustaining therapy and in decisions not to resuscitate, medical indications are of major import in formulating recommendations to the patient or to surrogates. Medical indications may be the primary basis for the physician's decision about appropriate treatment for those mentally incapacitated patients who have no surrogates. The ethical propriety of this practice will be examined in Chapter 2.

# Preferences of Patients

**2.0** This chapter discusses the second topic that is essential to the definition and resolution of an ethical problem in clinical medicine, namely, the preferences of patients. The first topic, medical indications, concerns the clinical judgment of the physician. Clinical judgment leads to a recommendation that is offered to the patient who must choose a preferred course. On some occasions, if the patient is incapable of choice, the recommendations are offered to the relatives or guardians. On other occasions, such as emergency care, physicians may be justified in acting on their own initiative. This chapter will discuss the issues associated with the expression or the absence of patient preferences in the following order: (1) the ethical, legal, clinical, and psychological significance of patient preferences; (2) informed consent; (3) decisional capacity; (4) unfamiliar beliefs; (5) refusal of treatment; (6) advanced directives; (7) surrogate decisions; (8) the uncooperative patient; (9) alternative medicine.

**The Significance of Patient Preferences.**   When there are medical indications for treatment, a physician normally proposes a treatment plan, which a competent patient may accept or refuse. An informed, competent patient's preference to accept or to refuse medically indicated treatment has ethical, legal, clinical, and psychological importance. Patient preferences are the ethical and legal nucleus of a patient-physician relationship; in most circumstances, the relationship can neither be initiated nor sustained unless the patient desires it. Even though the patient may need the assistance of a physician, physicians must remember that the patient, not the physician, has the primary legal and moral authority to establish the relationship. Further, knowledge of patient preferences is essential to good clinical care, since the patient's cooperation and satisfaction reflect the degree to which medical intervention fulfills the patient's choices, values and needs.

### 2.0.1   Clinical Significance of Patient Preferences

Patient preferences are clinically significant because patients who interact actively with their physicians to reach a shared health care decision have greater trust and loyalty in the doctor-patient relationship, cooperate more fully to implement the shared decision, express greater satisfaction with their health care, and most important, have now been shown to have better clinical outcomes in at least the following four chronic conditions: hypertension, non-insulin-dependent diabetes mellitus, peptic ulcer disease, and rheumatoid arthritis. Further research on the importance of patient involvement in decisions has shown that as medicine has become more effective, there are often several medically reasonable options for treating a particular problem, and each option is associated with different risks and benefits for the patient. For example, to avoid the risk of perioperative death, some patients with lung cancer may choose radiation therapy over surgery despite a lower five-year survival rate. Similarly, some patients may choose prophylactic mastectomy over watchful waiting when told they have a strong genetic susceptibility to breast cancer or may choose watchful waiting rather than surgery for symptomatic benign prostatic hypertrophy.

Rational patient choice is based both on medical indications and on patient preferences. Therefore, different patients may express quite different but entirely reasonable preferences when faced with the same medical indications. Recent research has also shown that some physicians are more likely than others to invite the expression of patient preferences and to encourage a "participatory decision-making style." It appears that health outcomes for patients with chronic diseases improve when patients ask questions, express opinions, and make their preferences known, and when physicians have a "participatory" rather than a "controlling" decision-making style. A participatory style is associated with primary care training, skill in interviewing which facilitates empathic listening and communication, and the opportunity to take time with patients. [Kaplan SH, Greenfield S, Ware JE. Assessing the effects of physician-patient interactions on the outcomes of chronic disease. *Medical Care* 1989; 27 (No.3 Supplement): S110–127; Kaplan SH, Greenfield S, Gandek B, Rogers WH, Ware JE. Characteristics of physicians with participatory decision-making styles. *Ann Intern Med* 1996; 124:497–504; More E, Milligan M eds. *The Empathic Practitioner.* New Brunswick, N.J. Rutgers University Press, 1995.]

### 2.0.2    Legal Significance: Self-Determination

Patient preferences are legally significant because the American legal system recognizes that each person has a fundamental right to control his or her own body and the right to be protected from unwanted intrusions or "unconsented touchings." An early judicial opinion on this matter states the principle quite frankly:

> Every human being of adult years and of sound mind has a right to determine what shall be done with his body. [Schloendorff v. Society of New York Hospital, 1914.]

A more recent leading case reiterates the principle:

> Anglo-American law starts with the premise of thoroughgoing self-determination. It follows that each man is considered to be master of his own body, and he may, if he be of sound mind, prohibit the performance of life-saving surgery or other medical treatment. [Natanson v. Kline, 1960.]

The legal requirement of explicit consent prior to specific treatment protects patients' legal right to control what is done to their own bodies. The documentation of the patient's consent also serves as a defense for the physician against a claim that the patient was coerced.

In addition, patient preferences are significant because the law has sometimes considered the patient-physician relationship to be a "fiduciary relationship," in which the fiduciary, in this case the physician, has an obligation to promote the best interests of persons who have entrusted themselves to the physician's care. The patient's consent initiates this relationship and sustains it by accepting the recommendations of the physician. The concept of fiduciary relationship is discussed at 4.0.4.

Finally, apart from clinical skill and carefulness, respect for patient preferences and a participatory style of dealing with patients appear to be the primary protection that physicians have against malpractice. Patients are much less inclined to bring legal action against such physicians.

### 2.0.3    Psychological Significance: Control

Patient preferences are psychologically significant because the ability to express preferences and have others respect them is crucial to a sense of personal worth. The patient, already threatened by disease, may have a vital need for some sense of control. Furthermore, if patient preferences are ignored or devalued, patients are likely to distrust and perhaps disregard physicians' recommendations. If patients are overtly or covertly uncooperative, the effectiveness of therapy is threatened. Furthermore, patient preferences are important because their expression may lead to the discovery of other factors—such as fears, fantasies, or unusual beliefs—that the physician should consider in dealing with the patient.

### 2.0.4    Policy Significance of Patient Preferences

Many surveys have shown that the public is concerned about the right to choose one's own physician, the right to choose one's system of care (fee-for-service or managed care), and the right to make one's own health care decisions. Further, recent studies show that, when faced with professional uncertainty about which of several options are best, patients often make conservative choices that reduce their own risk while at the same time decreasing health care costs. The inefficiency of provider-driven demand is countered by informed patient preferences. Thus, the hypothesis can be offered that policy encouraging a patient-centered approach that allows patients to indicate their preferences and to reach decisions with their physicians in a shared or participatory style would improve the efficiency and cost effectiveness of health care. Further study of this hypothesis is needed.

### 2.0.5    Ethical Significance: Autonomy

Patient preferences are ethically significant because they make explicit the value of personal autonomy that is deeply rooted in the ethics of our culture. Moral philosophers emphasize the principle of autonomy, the moral right to choose and follow one's own plan of life and action. Respect for autonomy is the moral attitude that disposes one to refrain from interference with others' autonomous beliefs and actions in the pursuit of their goals. Constraint of a person's free choices is morally permissible only when one person's preferences and actions seriously infringe on another's rights and welfare. The recognition of patient preferences respects the value of personal autonomy in medical care. In practice, however, many forces obstruct and limit the expression and appreciation of patient preferences. These forces—such as the compromised competence of the patient, disparity between practitioner's knowledge and that of the patient, the psychodynamics of the patient-physician relationship, the stress of illness—often make difficult the realization of respect for the autonomy of the patient. [EB: "Autonomy," I, 215–220; PBE: ch. 3; ME: ch. 2.]

### 2.0.6 Paternalism

One of the most common ethical issues raised by the principle of respect for autonomy is paternalism. This term refers to the practice of overriding or ignoring preferences of patients in order to benefit them or enhance their welfare. In essence, it consists in the judgment that beneficence takes priority over autonomy. Historically, the medical profession has endorsed paternalism; today, while still common, it is considered ethically suspect. Still, there are situations in which paternalistic behavior is ethically justified. These will be noted at various points in the subsequent pages. [EB: "Paternalism," IV, 1914–1920; PBE: "Paternalism: Conflicts Between Beneficence and Autonomy," 271–291; Childress, J: *Who Should Decide? Paternalism in Health Care*. New York: Oxford University Press, 1982.]

### 2.0.7 P The Preferences of the Child

As children become mature enough to articulate their preferences and reasons for them, they are entitled to increasing respect for these preferences. They are led toward responsible maturity by this respect, as well as by education. However, it is sometimes difficult to decide how much respect to afford a child's preferences, especially when these seem to be contrary to the child's welfare. It is also difficult to discern how rational these preferences are, because consequences and alternatives, as well as relative values, are often not perceived clearly by the child.

### 2.0.8 P Legal Consent of Minors

Minors, that is, persons who are younger than the statutory age of consent (age 18 in all states), may come to a physician on their own initiative. If their medical problem is not an emergency, such persons can be treated only with the consent of their parents (2.7.5 P). However, there are several exceptions.

(a) Almost all jurisdictions now have special provisions for the treatment of certain conditions without the consent of the minor's parents. These conditions are usually drug abuse and venereal disease (contraception, abortion, and mental illness are sometimes included, sometimes specifically excluded). Physicians should be aware of the provisions of the law in the jurisdiction in which they practice.

(b) The emancipated minor is a young person who lives independently of parents, physically, financially, or otherwise. Married minors, those in the armed forces or living away at college are considered emancipated. They may request treatment and be treated without parental consent.

(c) The legal concept of "mature minor" is increasingly invoked. A mature minor is one who is below statutory age and who is still dependent upon parents but who appears to make reasoned judgments. These young persons pose something of a quandary to the physician from whom they seek care. On the one hand, they appear able to decide for themselves; on the other hand, their parents remain legally responsible for them. Legal authorities conclude the physician may respond to their requests under the following conditions:

(i) The patient is at the age of discretion (15 years or older) and appears able to understand the procedure and its risks sufficiently to be able to give a genuinely informed consent.

(ii) The medical measures are taken for the patient's own benefit (i.e., not as a transplant donor or research subject).

(iii) The measures can be justified as necessary by medical opinion.

(iv) There is some good reason, including simple refusal by the minor to request it, why parental consent cannot be obtained.

A physician may treat a minor without parental consent if the minor is emancipated or if there is statutory authorization for certain sorts of treatment. If the minor does not fit either category but is capable of understanding and consent, the physician may treat under the conditions mentioned above. In the case of the mature minor, however, the physician should inquire, if possible, about the reasons for the young person's unwillingness to communicate with parents. Steps should be taken, if the minor is willing, to attempt reconciliation or to solve the problem in a mutually satisfactory manner. Confidentiality should be maintained. Physicians should note that confidentiality is often unintentionally breached by billing procedures.

Physicians who honor the requests of mature minors are at some theoretical legal risk. However, "no decisions can be found within the past 20 years in which a parent recovered damages, even in the absence of a minor treatment statute, for treatment of a child over the age of 15 without parental consent. [Holder A. *Legal Issues in Pediatrics and Adolescent Medicine.* New Haven: Yale University Press, 1985.]

A request for irreversible sterilization from a mature minor poses peculiar problems. There are statutory and regulatory prohibitions against sterilization of minors in certain federal programs and in many states. There is peril of a suit by parents and by the minor at a later date. There is good reason to assume that even a mature minor cannot comprehend the implications of this procedure. A physician confronted with this request should certainly explore the reasons behind the request and offer less radical alternatives. [EB: "Children," "Adolescents," I, 351–377, 63–71.]

**2.1**                          **INFORMED CONSENT**

The usual vehicle for the expression of patient preferences is the process of informed consent. It is a practical application of respect for the patient's autonomy. When a patient consults a physician for a suspected medical problem, the physician makes a diagnosis and recommends treatment. The physician explains these steps to the patient, giving the reason for the recommended treatment, the option of alternative treatments, and the benefits and burdens of all options. The patient understands the information, assesses the treatment choices, and expresses a preference for one of the options proposed by the physician. This ideal scenario captures the essence of the informed consent process. As an ethical basis for the patient-physician relationship, informed consent refers to an encounter characterized by mutual participation, respect, and shared decision-making. Informed consent should not designate a mechanical recitation of facts or a pro forma signature on a piece of paper. The phrase "I consented the patient," used too frequently by young clinicians, reveals a casual attitude toward informed consent.

Informed consent should represent a dialogue between physician and patient leading to agreement about the course of medical care. Informed consent establishes a reciprocal relationship or therapeutic alliance between physician and patient which includes, at its best, appropriate communication, good advice, mutual respect, and rational choices. Further, after initial consent to treatment has occurred, a continuing dialogue between patient and physician, based on the patient's continuing medical needs, reinforces the original consent. A properly negotiated informed consent benefits the physician as well as the patient: a therapeutic alliance is forged in which the physician's work is facilitated because the patient has realistic expectations about outcomes of treatment, is prepared for possible complications, and is more likely to be a willing collaborator in treatment. [EB: "Informed Consent," III, 1232–1270; PBE: "The Meaning and Justification of Informed Consent," 142–170; ME: ch. 7, 185–208; President's Commission. *Making Health Care Decisions*. Washington, D.C.: Government Printing Office, 1982; Appelbaum PS, Lidz CW, Meisel A. *Informed Consent: Legal Theory and Clinical Practice*. New York: Oxford University Press, 1987; Faden R, Beauchamp T. *A History and Theory of Informed Consent*. New York: Oxford University Press, 1986; Katz J. *The Silent World of Doctor and Patient*. New York: The Free Press, 1984.]

*EXAMPLE.*    Mr. Cure, the patient with pneumococcal meningitis, is told that he needs immediate antibiotic therapy. After he is informed of the nature of his disease, the benefits and burdens of treatment, and the possible consequences of nontreatment, he expresses his preference by consenting to the antibiotic therapy. A therapeutic alliance that is clinically, ethically, and emotionally satisfactory is formed and reinforced when the patient recovers.

*EXAMPLE.*    Mr. Cope is a 42-year-old man who was diagnosed as having insulin-dependent diabetes at age 21. Insulin was prescribed and a dietary regimen recommended. In the intervening years, he has complied with his dietary and medical regimen, but has experienced repeated episodes of ketoacidosis and hypoglycemia. His physician has regularly discussed with Mr. Cope the course of his disease, the treatment plan and inquired about his difficulties in coping with his condition.

*COMMENT:*    Example I exemplifies what might be called routine consent. The physician expresses clinical judgment by making recommendations to the patient regarding an appropriate course of care. The patient makes known his preference by presenting himself for diagnosis and treatment and by accepting, usually explicitly, the physicians' recommendations. Example II is also routine consent, but in a chronic disease. Mr. Cope's doctor was assiduous in informing and educating his patient. Mr. Cope accepted the treatment regimen, and his compliance with it shows his preferences. However, in chronic diseases, which often have variable courses, the patient may not be fully informed about, or aware of, the future implications of treatment or nontreatment. We shall see problems develop in both these cases in the following pages.

### 2.1.1   Informed Consent: Definition and Standard

Informed consent is defined as the willing acceptance of a medical intervention by a patient after adequate disclosure by the physician of the nature of the intervention, its risks, and benefits, as well as of alternatives with their risks and benefits. How should it be determined that a disclosure of information by a physician is adequate? One approach is to ask what a reasonable and prudent physician would tell a patient. This approach, the legal standard in some of the early informed consent cases, is increasingly being replaced by a new standard. The legal trend is to set as the standard what reasonable patients need to know to make rational decisions. The former standard affords greater discretion to the physician; the latter is more patient-centered. A third standard, sometimes called a "subjective" standard, is patient-specific. The question then is whether the information provided is specifically tailored to a particular patient's need for information and understanding. Although the law usually requires that the physician meet only the reasonable patient standard, a physician who engages in a participatory style of shared decision-making is likely to aspire to the requirements of a subjective standard. The reasonable person standard may be ethically sufficient, but the subjective standard is ethically ideal.

### 2.1.2   Scope of Disclosure

Many studies show that patients desire information from their physicians; many practitioners are aware that their patients appreciate information. In recent years, candid disclosure, even of "bad news," has become the norm. It is widely agreed that disclosure should include:

- The patient's current medical status, including the likely course if no treatment is provided
- The interventions that might improve prognosis, including a description and the risks and benefits of those procedures, as well as some estimation of probabilities and uncertainties associated with the interventions
  - A professional opinion about alternatives open to the patient
  - A recommendation based on the physician's best clinical judgment

In conveying this information, physicians should avoid technical terms, attempt to translate statistical data into everyday probabilities, ask whether the patient understands the information, and invite questions. Physicians are not obliged, as one court said, to give each patient "a mini-medical education." Still, physicians should strive to educate their patients about their specific medical needs and options.

## 2.1.3    Stringency

The moral and legal obligation of disclosure also varies in terms of the situation; it becomes more stringent and demanding as the treatment situation moves from emergency through elective to experimental. In some emergency situations, very little information can be provided. Any attempt to inform may be at the price of precious time. Ethically and legally, information can be curtailed in emergencies (2.7.3). When treatment is elective, much more information should be provided. Finally, detailed and thorough information should accompany any invitation to participate in research, particularly if the research maneuver is not directed to the patient's therapy (4.6).

## 2.1.4    Comprehension

The phrase "informed consent" stresses the giving of information. Most legal discussions of informed consent emphasize the amount and kind of information the doctor provides. Consent forms list risks and benefits. However, the comprehension of the patient is as fully important as the providing of information. Some studies and many anecdotes suggest that the comprehension by patients of medical information is not outstanding. At the same time, studies suggest that methods of communication are poor and that little effort is made to overcome barriers to comprehension. The physician has an ethical obligation to make reasonable efforts to assure comprehension. Explanations should be given clearly and simply; questions should be asked to assess understanding. Written instructions or printed materials should be provided. Video or computer programs should be provided to guide patients who face complicated decisions, such as choosing between options for treatment of breast cancer or prostate cancer. Educational programs for patients with chronic disease should be arranged.

## 2.1.5 Difficulties with Informed Consent

The process of informed consent is not easy. Physicians may be trapped in technical language, troubled by the uncertainty intrinsic to all medical information, worried about harming or alarming the patient, hurried and pressed by multiple obligations. Patients may be limited in understanding, inattentive and distracted, or overcome by fear and anxiety. Patients may believe that decisions are the physician's prerogative; physicians may not appreciate the rationale for the patient's participation. Thus, many physicians feel the informed consent requirement imposes upon them an undesirable and perhaps impossible task: undesirable because adequately informing a patient takes too long and might create unnecessary anxiety, impossible because no medically uneducated and clinically inexperienced patient can truly grasp the significance of the information the physician must disclose. Even physicians, when they are patients, may not comprehend information germane to their own illness. Selective hearing because of denial, fear, or preoccupation with illness may account for failure to take in what one might otherwise understand. For these reasons physicians sometimes dismiss the informed consent requirement as a meaningless but bureaucratically necessary ritual. This is a sadly limited view of the ethical purpose of informed consent. Informed consent is not merely pushing information at a patient. It is an opportunity to initiate dialogue between physicians and their patients in which both attempt to arrive at a mutually satisfactory course of action. Informed consent should result in shared decision-making. The process, while difficult, is not impossible and is always open to improvement. Finally, the dialogue between physicians and patients is not only inhibited by limitations of physician communication and patient comprehension: it is limited by the inability of many physicians to listen carefully to their patients' words and the emotions underlying them.

## 2.2                          DECISIONAL CAPACITY

Consent to treatment is complicated not only by the difficulties of disclosure but also because some patients lack the mental capacity to understand or to make choices. The law often uses the terms "competence" and "incompetence" to designate whether persons have the legal authority to make personal choices, such as managing their finances or making health care decisions. Judges alone have the right to rule that a person is legally incompetent. Medical practitioners may encounter legally competent patients who appear to have their mental capacities compromised by illness, anxiety, pain, or hospitalization. We refer to this clinical situation as decisional capacity or incapacity, in order to distinguish it from the legal determination of competency. It is necessary to assess decisional capacity as an essential part of the informed consent process. [EB: "Competence," I, 445–450; PBE, "Competence and Autonomous Choice," 132–141; ME: ch. 10, 292–307.]

### 2.2.1  The Concept of Decisional Capacity

In a medical setting a patient's capacity to consent to or refuse care requires at least an ability to understand relevant information, to appreciate the medical situation and its possible consequences, to communicate a choice, and to engage in rational deliberation about one's own values in relation to the physician's recommendations about treatment options. For patients who obviously possess the relevant abilities, capacity to decide for themselves is not seriously questioned. Their right to make their own decisions based on their preferences should be respected. Patients who clearly lack these abilities, e.g., because they are unconscious or are manifestly disoriented and delusional, fall below the threshold of decisional capacity. For them a surrogate decision-maker is required. For some patients, however, it may be uncertain whether they fall above or below the threshold for decisional capacity. These are the problematic cases.

### 2.2.2  Determining Decisional Capacity

The first step in making a determination of capacity is to engage in ordinary conversation with the patient, to observe the patient's behavior, and to talk with third parties—staff, family, or friends. But clinicians should be alert to clues that apparent competence is illusory. Paranoid patients appear normal until certain questions trigger a delusional belief system. Patients who too quickly agree to a physician's recommendations may not really understand what is being proposed. The mental capacity of patients who refuse a low-risk, high-benefit treatment without which they face serious injury or death is naturally suspect.

Decisional capacity refers to the specific acts of comprehending, evaluating, and choosing among realistic options. Physicians, attempting to assess a patient's decisional capacity, should not depend on global descriptions such as schizophrenia, depression, or dementia. What is important is how these general psychological states and psychiatric diagnoses affect the patient's ability to understand and choose in a particular situation. Many persons with psychopathologies retain the ability to make reasonable decisions about particular choices that face them.

When a clinician doubts a patient's decisional capacity to make particular choices, formal and informal tests for cognitive functioning, psychiatric disorders, or organic conditions that may affect decisional capacity can be utilized. However, no single test is sufficient to capture the complex concept of decisional capacity in a clinical setting. Some conditions, such as an affective state of anxiety or depression, may be transitory or reversible with psychiatric intervention. Other conditions, such as drug-induced confusion, may be resolved by titrating medication properly. But some problems, such as inability to understand simple explanations of facts or fixed delusions, may be impossible to remedy. In cases where determination of capacity is problematic, clinicians should seek consultation from local resources—psychiatric liaison services, hospital risk managers, attorneys, ethics committees, or consultants. If there is sufficient clinical evidence that a patient is decisionally incapacitated, an appropriate surrogate decision-maker assumes authority, as explained in 2.7. It is important to realize that even a patient who might be seriously incapacitated might nevertheless retain the ability to designate a surrogate.

**Case I.** Mr. Cope, the 42-year-old man with insulin-dependent diabetes, is brought by his wife to the emergency department with complaints of a flulike syndrome with fever, myalgias, anorexia, vomiting, and gradually developing stupor. His wife reports that, for two days, Mr. Cope has been unable to eat, drink, or take oral medications. On the day prior to presentation, he also did not take his morning or evening insulin. On evaluation in the emergency department, he is stuporous but opens his eyes when people shout his name or pinch his skin. Vital signs are: temperature 39.1°C, BP 100/70, pulse 110 and regular, and respirations 24–26 with deep Kussmaul respirations. Other positive physical findings include prominent basilar rales noted in the right lung posteriorly, and the right foot was cool compared with the left. The right femoral artery was palpable but diminished compared with the left; a bruit was noted over the right femoral; no pulses were felt in the right leg distal to the femoral. Initial laboratory studies confirmed the clinical impression of acute right lower lobe pneumonia and diabetic ketoacidosis, with glucose 754, sodium 124, potassium 5.6, chloride 91 $CO_2$ 12, BUN 60, creatinine 2.2, and arterial blood gases of pH 7.10, $P_{O_2}$ of 65 and $P_{CO_2}$ of 26. Based on these findings, the physicians proposed vigorous treatment for the diabetic ketoacidosis with intravenous insulin and fluid and electrolyte repletion. In addition, although the right lower lobe pneumonia was thought to be viral, the physicians recommended antibiotics to cover the possibility of a community-acquired bacterial pneumonia or an aspiration pneumonia. Although Mr. Cope was generally somnolent and stuporous, he awoke while the IV was being inserted and stated loudly: "Leave me alone. No needles and no hospital. I'm OK." His wife urged the medical team to disregard the patient's statements: "He is not himself."

*COMMENT:* We agree with Mrs. Cope's assessment of the situation. Mr. Cope has an acute crisis (ketoacedosis and pneumonia) superimposed on a chronic disease (type I diabetes) and he now presents with progressive stupor over a two-day period. At this time, he clearly lacks decisional capacity, although he was capable of making decisions two days earlier, before the onset of his illness, and is likely to be able to make his own decisions again when he recovers from the ketoacidosis, probably within the next 24 hours. At this moment, it would be unethical to be guided by the shouts of an individual who lacks decision-making capacity. The physicians would be correct to be guided by the wishes of the patient's surrogate, his wife, and to treat over the objections of Mr. Cope. Issues associated with surrogate decision-making are discussed at 2.7. We shall encounter another problem with Mr. Cope at 2.5.

**Case II.** In the case presented at 1.0 and 2.1, Mr. Cure has symptoms suggestive of bacterial meningitis. He is informed that he needs immediate hospitalization and administration of antibiotics. He refuses treatment and says he wants to go home. The physician explains the extreme dangers of going untreated and the minimal risks of treatment. The young man persists in his refusal. Apart from this strange demand, he exhibits no evidence of mental derangement or altered mental status.

*COMMENT:*   There is no overt clinical evidence to support a judgment that Mr. Cure is incapacitated. The physician might presume altered mental status due to fever or metabolic disturbance, but mere presumption, in the absence of affective and behavioral clues, is inadequate to justify a conclusion that he is incapacitated. Physicians sometimes assume that any refusal of lifesaving treatment is "crazy" and suppose the person to be incompetent. Refusal of treatment should not, in and of itself, be considered the act of an incapacitated person. There must be clinical evidence or solid medical reason to justify the judgment of incapacity. Is it ethically permissible to treat against his will a patient with a life-threatening condition whose capacity to choose appears intact? The case is further discussed under Enigmatic Refusal (2.5.3).

**Case III.**   Mrs. D., 77 years old, is brought to the emergency department by a neighbor. Her left foot is gangrenous. She has lived alone for the last 12 years and is known by neighbors and by her doctor to be intelligent and fiercely independent. Her mental abilities are relatively intact, but she is becoming quite forgetful and is sometimes confused. On her last two visits to her doctor, she consistently called him by the name of her former physician, who is now dead. On being told that the best medical option for her problem is amputation, she adamantly refuses, although she insists she is aware of the consequences and accepts them. She calmly tells her doctor (whom she again calls by the wrong name) that she wants to be buried whole. He considers whether to seek judicial authority to treat.

*COMMENT:*   Mrs. D.'s mild dementia casts doubt on her ability to make an autonomous judgment. However, even persons whose mental performance is somewhat abnormal should not thereby be disqualified as decision-makers. Persons might not be well oriented to time and place and still understand the issue confronting them. The central test of competence is the evidence that a person seems to understand the nature of the issue and the consequences of the choice he or she is making. It is also possible to place any choice in the context of a person's own life history and values and ask whether the particular choice seems consistent with these. This is sometimes called the "authenticity" of the choice. While ethicists argue over this as a criterion of mental capacity, it can often be a helpful clinical guide in evaluating the autonomy of the choice.

*RECOMMENDATION:* Mrs. D.'s clear assertions, as well as the broader evidence of her life and values, suggest that she has adequate decisional capacity to make an autonomous choice. Her physician should not seek a judicial determination of incompetence, unless genuine doubt exists about her decisional capacity. Treatment of Mrs. D. should be limited to appropriate medical management. It is appropriate to attempt gentle persuasion to accept amputation, but no undue pressure or coercion should be used.

**Case III (Continued).**   Mrs. D. presents to the ER as described above. However, in this version of the case, she adamantly denies that she has any medical problem. Although the toes of her left foot are necrotic and gangrenous tissue extends above the ankle, she insists that she is in perfect health and has been taking her daily walk every day, even this morning. Her neighbor affirms that Mrs. D. has been housebound for at least a week, which had led her to drop in to see whether there was a problem.

*RECOMMENDATION:* In this version, Mrs. D. seems decisionally incapacitated. She is denying her infirmity and her need for care and appears to be delusional. In Mrs. D.'s best interests (2.7, 3.0.3), the appointment of a surrogate should be sought and a decision about surgery considered.

## 2.2.3   Evaluating Decisional Capacity in Relation to the Need for Intervention

Usually a patient's capacity is not seriously questioned unless the patient decides to refuse or discontinue treatment. In such situations, tests of capacity to consent might be applied. These tests can range from the simplest tests of mental status available to any physician to the more sophisticated evaluations applied by a psychiatrist or clinical psychologist. It has been suggested that the stringency of the test should vary with the seriousness of the disease and urgency for treatment; the standard of capacity required for decision-making varies with the extent and probability of risk, with the extent and probability of benefit, and with consent or refusal. For example, a patient might need to meet a low standard of capacity to consent to a procedure with substantial, highly probable benefits and minimal, low-probability risk, but a higher standard of competence should be required to refuse the same treatment. [Drane JF. Competency to give informed consent. *JAMA* 1984; 252:925–927; Applebaum PS, Grisso T. Assessing patient's capacities to consent to treatment. *NEJM* 1988; 319:1635; Lo B. Assessing decision-making capacity. *Am J Law Med* 1990; 18:192; Applebaum PS, Grisso T. Comparison of standards for assessing patients' capacities to make treatment decisions. *Am J Psychiatry* 1995; 152:1033–1037.]

**2.2.4   Waxing and Waning Capacity**

Certain pathological conditions, such as organic brain syndrome, are characterized by a movement in and out of mental clarity. Similarly, a patient's mental capacity often changes during the day, as in the so-called sundowner syndrome. Thus, a patient may at one time appear clear and oriented but later be assessed as incapacitated.

*EXAMPLE.* Mrs. Care, with MS, is now hospitalized. In the morning she is able to converse intelligibly with doctors, nurses, and family. In the afternoon she confabulates and is disoriented to place and time. In both conditions she expresses various preferences about care, which are sometimes contradictory. In particular, when questioned about surgical placement of a tube to prevent aspiration, she says no in the morning and, in the afternoon, speaks confusedly and repeatedly about having the tube placed.

*RECOMMENDATION:* This waxing and waning is itself the manifestation of pathology. The patient should be considered to have impaired capacity. The expression of preferences in such a state should not be considered determinative, unless there is consistency in the preferences expressed during periods of clarity.

**2.3            UNFAMILIAR BELIEFS:**
**RELIGIOUS AND CULTURAL DIVERSITY**

Certain religious denominations hold beliefs about health, sickness, and medical care that may be unfamiliar to providers; sometimes such beliefs will influence the patient's preferences about care in ways that providers might consider imprudent or dangerous. Similarly, persons from cultural traditions differing from the prevailing culture may view the medical practices of the prevailing culture as strange and even repugnant. In both cases, providers will be faced with the problem of reconciling a clinical judgment that seems reasonable to them, and even an ethical judgment that seems obligatory, with a patient's preference for a different course of action. The appropriate response to such situations will be treated under the two topics where they usually arise: truthful disclosure (2.4) and competent refusal of treatment (2.5), and also under the role of family in making decisions (4.1.3). Some general comments are appropriate here:

(a) Unfamiliarity with beliefs and customs of others may lead providers to question the mental capacity of the patient. Physicians and nurses may judge as "crazy" anyone refusing standard medical treatment. The mere fact of adherence to an unusual belief is not, in and of itself, evidence of incapacity. In the absence of clinical signs of incapacity, such persons should be considered capable of choice.

(b) In institutions where there is a high volume of patients from a particular religious or cultural tradition, providers must educate themselves about the beliefs of those patients, have competent translators available, and make use of mediators, such as clergy or educated persons who can explain the beliefs and communicate with those who hold them. At the same time, the mere fact that a person speaks the same language or comes from the same country or religion as the patient does not guarantee competence as a translator or intermediary. Also, providers should be careful to avoid cultural stereotypes: there are individuals from particular cultures who depart, in their values, preferences and life-style, from the predominant mode of their cultures.

(c) To the extent possible, negotiation should attempt to find a course acceptable to the patient and provider alike. It is first necessary to discover the common goals that are sought by the patient and the physician and to settle on mutually acceptable strategies to attain those goals. The ethical response to a genuine conflict in an essential matter is dependent on the circumstances of the case and will be discussed below, under truthful communication and refusal of care. Cases in which cultural differences play a significant role are found in 2.5 and 4.1.3. [Special Section. Cross-cultural perspectives in health care. *Cambridge Quarterly of Healthcare Ethics* 1994; 3 (3); Cultural differences in bioethics. *J Clin Ethics* 1993; 4(2); Jecker NS, Carrese JA, Pearlman RA. Caring for patients in cross-cultural settings. *Hastings Center Report* 1995; 25 (1):6–14; Cross-cultural medicine. (Special issue). *West J Med* 1992; 157 (3); Galanti GA. *Caring for Patients from Different Cultures.* Philadelphia: University of Pennsylvania Press, 1991.]

**2.4**                    **TRUTHFUL COMMUNICATION**

Communications between physicians and patients should be truthful, that is, statements should be in accord with facts. If the facts are uncertain, that uncertainty should be acknowledged. Deception, by stating what is untrue or by omitting what is true, should be avoided. These ethical principles govern all human communication. However, in the communication between patients and physicians, certain ethical problems arise about truthfulness. Does the patient really want to know the truth? What if the truth, once known, causes harm? Might not deception help by providing hope? In the past, medical ethics has given ambiguous answers to these questions: while some authors favored truthfulness, others recommended beneficent deception. More recently, with the prominence of the doctrine of informed consent, truthfulness has been commended as the ethical course of action. [EB: "Information Disclosure," III, 1221–1232; PBE, "Veracity," 395–406; Bok S. *Lying: Moral Choice in Public and Private Life.* New York: Pantheon, 1978.]

**Case I.**   Mr. R.S., a 65-year-old man, comes to his physician with complaints of weight loss and mild abdominal discomfort. The patient, whom the physician knows well, has just retired from a busy career and has made plans for a round-the-world tour with his wife. Studies reveal mild elevation in liver functions and a questionable mass in the tail of the pancreas. At the beginning of his interview with his physician to discuss the test results, Mr. R.S. remarks, "Doc, I hope you don't have any bad news for me. We've got big plans." Ordinarily, a needle biopsy of the pancreas to confirm pancreatic cancer would be the next step. The physician wonders whether he should put this off until Mr. R.S. returns from his trip. Should the physician's concern that Mr. R.S. may have pancreatic cancer be revealed to him at this time?

*COMMENT:*   In recent years, commentators on this problem have moved away from the ambiguous position of traditional medical ethics, which favored beneficent deception, toward a strong assertion of the patient's right to the truth. Their arguments are:

(a) There is a strong moral duty to tell the truth that is not easily overridden by speculation about possible harms.

(b) The patient has a need for the truth if he or she is to make rational decisions about actions and plans for life.

(c) Concealment of the truth is likely to undermine the patient-physician relationship. In case of serious illness, it is particularly important that this relationship be strong.

(d) Tolerance of concealment by the profession may undermine the trust that the public should have in the profession. Widespread belief that physicians are not truthful would create an atmosphere in which persons who fear being deceived would not seek needed care.

(e) Suspicion on the part of the physician that truthful disclosure would be harmful to the patient may be founded on little or no evidence. It may arise more from the physician's own uneasiness at being a "bearer of bad news" than from the patient's inability to accept the information.

(f) Recent studies have shown that most patients with diagnoses of serious illness wish to know the diagnosis. Similarly, recent studies are unable to document harmful effects of full disclosure.

(g) The law has traditionally allowed physicians a so-called therapeutic privilege to withhold information under certain circumstances. However, those circumstances are very narrow: "when a doctor can prove by a preponderance of the evidence he relied upon facts which would demonstrate to a reasonable man that the disclosure would have so seriously upset the patient that the patient would not have been able to dispassionately weigh the risks of refusing to undergo the recommended treatment." (Cobbs v. Grant, Cal. Sup. Ct., 1972.)

*RECOMMENDATION:* Mr. R.S. should be told the truth: he probably has cancer of the pancreas. The considerations in favor of truthful disclosure are, in our opinion, conclusive in establishing a strong ethical obligation on the physician to tell the truth to patients about their diagnosis and its treatment. The following are relevant:

(a) Speaking truthfully means relating the facts of the situation. This does not preclude a manner of relating the facts that is measured to perceptions of the hearer's emotional resilience and intellectual comprehension. The truth may be "brutal," but telling of it should not be. Measured and sensitive disclosure is demanded by respect for the autonomy and the sensitivities of the patient. It reinforces the patient's ability to deliberate and choose; it does not overwhelm this ability.

(b) Truthful disclosure has implications for Mr. R.S.'s plans. Further diagnostic studies might be done, appropriate treatments chosen. The trip might be delayed or canceled. Estate planning might be considered. Mr. R.S. should have the opportunity to reflect on these matters and to take control of his future. If some facts have no implications for the patient's deliberation and choices, they need not be revealed.

**Case II.** Mr. S.P., a 55-year-old teacher, has had chest pains and several fainting spells during the past three months. He reluctantly visits a physician at his wife's urging. He is very nervous and anxious and says to the physician at the beginning of the interview that he abhors doctors and hospitals. On physical examination, he has classic signs of tight aortic stenosis. The physician wishes to recommend cardiac catheterization. However, given his impression of this patient, he is worried lest full disclosure of the risks of catheterization would lead the patient to refuse the procedure.

*COMMENT:* In this case, the anticipated harm is much more specific and dangerous than the harm contemplated in Case I. Hesitation about revealing the risks of a diagnostic or therapeutic procedure is based on the fear the patient will make a judgment detrimental to health and life. Also, in this case there is better reason to suspect this patient will react badly to the information than the patient in Case I.

*RECOMMENDATION:* The arguments in favor of truthful disclosure apply equally to this case and to Case I. Whether or not catheterization is accepted, the patient will need further medical care. This patient needs, above all, the benefits of a good and trusting relationship with a competent physician. Honesty is more likely to create that relationship than deception. Also, the physician's fears about the patient's refusal may be exaggerated. In addition, studies indicate that almost all patients desire disclosure. Finally, the physician might be concerned about the family's reaction if Mr. S.P. died unexpectedly during catheterization.

**Case III.** A person who donates blood for a relative is found to be positive for HIV antibody. The blood is discarded and the donor's name registered as "deferred." Should the donor be informed?

*RECOMMENDATION:* The donor should be informed and counseled. Further confirmatory testing is advisable. Since there is a risk of infectivity and there is a chance that information about behavior may reduce that risk, the person has the right to this information and to education about HIV infection. In addition, new treatment options for asymptomatic patients with HIV infection provide another reason to inform donors of their HIV status.

**Case IV.** A traditional Navajo man, 58 years old, is brought by his daughter to a community hospital which is authorized by the Indian Health Service to serve Native American patients. He is suffering severe angina. Studies show that he is a candidate for cardiac bypass surgery. The surgeon discusses the risks of surgery and says, as is his custom, that there is a slight risk that the patient may not wake up from surgery. The patient listened silently, returned home and refused to return to the hospital. His daughter, who is a trained nurse, explained, "The surgeon's words were very routine for him, but for my Dad it was like a death sentence." [Carrese JA, Rhodes LA. Western bioethics on the Navajo Reservation. *JAMA* 1995; 274:826–829.]

*COMMENT:* In Navajo culture, language has the power to shape reality. Thus, the explanation of possible risks is a prediction that the undesirable events are likely to occur. In that culture, persons are accustomed to speak always in positive ways and to avoid speaking about evil or harmful things. The usual practice of informed consent, which requires the disclosure of risks and adverse effects, can cause distress and drive patients away from needed care. Similar reservations about the frankness of informed consent are found in other cultures. This issue will be discussed again in Chapter 4, where we treat the role of the family (4.1.3).

*RECOMMENDATION:* Physicians who understand this feature of Navajo life should shape their discussions in accord with the expectations of the patient. The omission of negative information, even though it would be unethical in dealing with a non-Navajo patient, is appropriate. This ethical advice rests on the fundamental value that underlies the rule of informed consent, namely, respect for persons, which requires that persons be respected, not as abstract individuals, but as formed within the values of their cultures.

## 2.4.1 Completeness of Disclosure

Disclosure of options for treatment of a patient's condition should be complete, including the options which the physician recommends and also other options which the physician may believe are less desirable but which are still medically reasonable. In so doing, the physician may make it clear why he or she considers these other options less desirable. However, it might be asked whether the obligation of truthful disclosure requires telling a patient about even those interventions that are not medically reasonable, but which a patient may wish to consider.

**Case I.** A 41-year-old woman has a breast biopsy that reveals cancer. The physician knows that this patient has a history of noncompliance and cancellation of medical appointments. In light of this, the physician believes that the best treatment approach would be a modified radical mastectomy. Should he also describe an alternative approach that includes lumpectomy, breast reconstruction, and a five-week course of radiation therapy? The physician is concerned that following a lumpectomy the patient may not keep her appointments.

*RECOMMENDATION:* The entire range of options should be explained with a careful delineation of the risks and benefits of each. There is no ethical prohibition against making a strong argument in favor of the option the physician considers best. Persuasion, however, should leave the patient free to choose, even if the physician believes she may choose the less effective option. Ultimately the patient must make decisions about breast surgery and keeping appointments. The physician must provide the patient with information and encourage her to complete whatever form of treatment she elects to receive.

## 2.4.2 Placebos

Placebo is defined as a substance given in the form of medicine but lacking specific activity for the condition being treated. This must be distinguished from the "placebo effect," which is the psychological, physiological, or psychophysiological effect of any medication given with therapeutic intent, but which is independent of any actual pharmacological effects. The placebo effect is known to take place as the result of many different influences: faith in the physician, administration of a medicine that the physician believes to be effective pharmacologically but is not, or actions of the physicians that are not in themselves therapeutic, such as taking a history or performing a diagnostic test. Thus, the placebo effect usually occurs without deliberate deception. In this broader sense, the placebo effect is a significant feature of medical practice, and the supposed benefits of a placebo treatment appear to depend on the qualities of the patient-physician relationship.

The problem of deception arises when the physician knows that the intervention does not have the objective properties necessary for efficacy and when the patient is kept ignorant of this fact. Examples are: monthly shots of vitamin $B_{12}$ for fatigue without a diagnosis of pernicious anemia; penicillin administered for a viral sore throat. In some cases, the deception is an outright moral offense, motivated solely by the desire to keep the patient's fees or to "get the patient off my back"; in other cases, placebo deception may raise a genuine ethical question. The duty not to deceive seems to conflict with the duty to benefit without doing harm.

It should be noted that placebo agents are now commonly used in controlled clinical trials of therapy for non-life-threatening conditions. Research subjects are informed that they will be randomized and may receive either an active drug or an inert substance. There is no deception involved and this practice is certainly ethical. [EB: "Placebo," IV, 1951–1953; PBE: "Intentional Non-disclosure," 150–153; Brody H. The lie that heals: the ethics of giving placebos. *Ann Intern Med* 1982; 97:112.]

**Case I.** A 73-year-old widow lives with her son. He brings her to a physician because she has become extremely lethargic and often confused. The physician determines that, after being widowed two years before, she had difficulty sleeping and had been prescribed hypnotics and that she is now addicted. The physician determines the best course would be to withdraw her from her present medication by a trial on placebos.

**Case II.** A 62-year-old man has had a total proctocolectomy and ileostomy for colonic cancer. There is no evidence of remaining tumor; the wound is healing well, and the ileostomy is functioning. On the eighth day after surgery, he complains of crampy abdominal pain and requests medication. The physician first prescribes antispasmodic drugs, but the patient's complaints persist. The patient requests morphine, which had relieved his postoperative pain. The physician is reluctant to prescribe opiates because repeated studies suggest that the pain is psychological and the physician knows that opiates will cause constipation. She contemplates a trial of placebo.

*COMMENT:* Any situation in which placebo use involves deliberate deception should be viewed as ethically problematic. The strong moral obligations of truthfulness and honesty prohibit deception; the danger to the patient-physician relationship advises against it. In those situations, however, when deceptive placebo use seems indicated, its ethical use would require at least the following conditions: (1) the condition to be treated should be known as one that has high response rates to placebo, for example, mild mental depression or postoperative pain; (2) the alternative to placebo is either continued illness or the use of a drug with known toxicity, for example, hypnotics as in Case I or morphine in Case II; (3) the patient wishes to be treated and cured, if possible; (4) the patient insists on a prescription.

*RECOMMENDATION:* The use of a placebo in Case I is not justified. The patient is not demanding medication. The problem of addiction should be confronted directly. There will be ample opportunity to develop a good relationship with this patient. Subsequent discovery of deception might undermine this relationship. Use of placebo in Case II is tempting but not ethically justifiable. In favor of placebo use, the patient is demanding relief. Morphine has adverse side effects. A short trial of placebo may be effective in relieving pain and avoiding the harm associated with opioids. However, explanation may be as effective as placebo use. The deceptive placebo can destroy the trust that creates the important and therapeutic "placebo effect" and can undermine the patient's confidence in the physician. A participatory style of decision-making is based on honest communication. Thus, even though we believe that placebo use might be theoretically justifiable, under the conditions expressed above, we doubt that such use is prudent in practice.

## 2.5 COMPETENT REFUSAL OF TREATMENT

Persons who are informed and are competent sometimes refuse recommended treatment. When the treatment is elective, ethical problems are unlikely. However, if care is judged necessary to save life or manage serious disease, physicians may be confronted with an ethical problem: Does the physician's responsibility to help the patient ever override the patient's freedom? Refusal of care by a competent and informed adult should be respected, even if that refusal leads to serious harm to the individual. This is ethically supported by the principle of autonomy and legally supported by American law. The patient's refusal of well-founded recommendations is often difficult for the conscientious physician to accept. It is made more difficult if the patient's refusal, while competent, seems irrational, that is, deliberately contrary to the patient's own welfare.

**Case I.** Ms. T.O. is a 64-year-old surgical nurse. Five years ago she had a resection of a stage I infiltrating ductal carcinoma. She visits her physician after discovering a mass in the contralateral breast and noting axillary swelling. Studies reveal stage II breast cancer with involved nodes. Following surgery, 10/16 nodes were positive. Chemotherapy and radiation are recommended and Ms. T.O. is told that the statistics for her condition suggest that, with treatment, she can expect a disease-free survival rate at ten years of 50 percent; without treatment, she has a 10 percent chance. She accepts chemotherapy, but after the first course, during which she has experienced significant toxicity, she informs her physician that she no longer wants any treatment. After extensive discussions with her physician and with her two daughters, she reaffirms her refusal of medical care.

**Case II.** Mr. S.P. has cardiac symptoms that indicate the need for coronary angiography. On hearing his physician explain the benefits and risks of this procedure, he decides he does not want it.

*RECOMMENDATION:* Ms. T.O. makes a competent refusal of treatment. She is very well informed and there is no evidence of any mental incapacitation. Even though the physician might consider the chances for prolonging disease-free survival good, Ms. T.O. values her risks and chances differently. Her refusal should be respected. Mr. S.P. is also competent. His refusal, even though it seems contrary to his interests, from the point of view of his ability to anticipate his health needs, is an expression of his autonomy. It must be respected. That respect, however, also should encourage the physician to explore more fully the reasons for the refusal and to attempt to educate and persuade. An early follow-up visit should be scheduled for both patients to assure them that their physician remains supportive and concerned to help them deal with the consequences of their decision.

**Case III.** We have seen Mr. Cope (2.2.2) admitted to the hospital for treatment of diabetic ketoacidosis with insulin, fluids, electrolytes, and antibiotics. That treatment was initiated over his objections, but on the authorization of his surrogate, Mrs. Cope, who was advised that his objections were the result of diabetic encephalopathy. After 24 hours, he awakens, talks appropriately with his family, recognizes and greets his physician. He does not remember having been brought to the emergency department. He now complains to the nurse and physician about pain in his right foot and wonders whether the foot was injured inadvertently when he was unresponsive and brought to the emergency department. Examination of the foot reveals that it is cold and mottled in color compared with the left foot, and no pulses can be felt in the right leg distal to the right femoral artery. A vascular surgery consultation confirms by Doppler study that there is an abrupt loss of pulses distal to the femoral artery and recommends an emergency arteriogram to determine if the patient has an embolic or thrombotic occlusion in the femoral system that may be treatable with angioplasty or embolectomy. This would prevent gangrene from developing in the right foot and leg and possibly prevent the need for amputation. After Mr. Cope is told the benefits and risks of the arteriogram, including the possible worsening of renal function, he declines to consent to arteriography. The surgeons explain to him that they cannot do angioplasty unless they know what vessel is involved and, further, that it is very difficult, almost impossible, to perform exploratory vascular surgery without knowing in advance the site of the arterial occlusion. They warn the patient that he faces a greater risk of losing his leg than a risk of losing renal function. Mr. Cope participates in these discussions, asking appropriate questions and acknowledging the doctors' comments. He then declines again to have the arteriography.

*COMMENT:* Although 24 hours ago, Mr. Cope was clearly decisionally incapacitated, and was properly treated for pneumonia and ketoacidosis, despite his insistence to be left alone, the current situation is entirely different. He has now regained decisional capacity, is able to understand the situation, can take account of risks and benefits, and make up his mind. His physician, nurses, and the consulting vascular surgeon agree that he has made a bad decision—that the low risk of worsening his renal function is more than compensated for by the substantial benefit of saving his leg. Mr. Cope does not agree. His family is divided, some siding with the doctors and some with Mr. Cope.

*RECOMMENDATION:*   Mr. Cope's decision must be respected. Efforts can be made to persuade him otherwise; time can be given for reconsideration. Still, Mr. Cope shows no signs of incapacitation and has the legal and moral right to make the decision that seems to him suitable. That decision may not be the right one from the viewpoint of medical indications, but law and ethics require respect for the patient's preferences in such circumstances.

### 2.5.1   Refusal on Grounds of Unfamiliar Belief

We noted the problem of evaluating unusual beliefs (2.3). Persons who hold unusual beliefs sometimes refuse medical recommendations.

**Case.**   Mr. G. comes to a physician for treatment of peptic ulcer. He says he is a Jehovah's Witness. He is a firm believer and knows his disease is one that may eventually require administration of blood. He quotes the biblical passage on which he bases his belief about blood transfusion not being utilized: "That ye abstain from meats offered to idols and from blood . . ." (Acts 15:28). The physician inquires of her Episcopal clergyman about the interpretation of this passage. He reports, after some research, that no Christian denomination except the Jehovah's Witnesses takes it to prohibit transfusion. The physician considers her patient's preferences impose an inferior standard of care. She wonders whether she should accept this patient under her care.

*COMMENT:*   As a general principle, the unusual beliefs and choices of other persons should be tolerated if they pose no threat to other parties. The patient's preferences should be respected, even though they appear mistaken to others.

(a) Jehovah's Witnesses cannot be considered incapacitated to make choices unless there is clinical evidence of such incapacity. This evidence should be developed as rigorously as for any other case of suspected decisional incapacity. On the contrary, these persons are usually quite clear about their belief and its consequences. It is a prominent part of their faith, insistently taught and discussed. Thus, while others may consider it irrational, adherence is not, in itself, a sign of incompetence.

(b) Courts have, in recent years, upheld the legal right of Jehovah's Witnesses to refuse lifesaving transfusions. If, however, unusual beliefs pose a threat to others it is ethically permissible and may be obligatory to prevent harm by means commensurate with the imminence of the threat and the seriousness of the harm. Thus, courts have consistently intervened to order blood transfusions for the minor children of Jehovah's Witnesses. Courts were once inclined to order an adult transfused for the sake of the adult's minor children but will now rarely do so, since alternative care for children is usually available.

(c) Refusal of blood transfusion differs in a significant way from refusal of all therapy or of recommended treatments. The Jehovah's Witnesses acknowledge the reality of their illness and desire to be cured or cared for; they simply reject one modality of care. Physicians may feel this limitation involves them in substandard and incompetent medical care.

(d) The physician's inquiry about the interpretation of the biblical passage is interesting. Presumably, she would feel more comfortable with a belief she knew to be part of her own religious tradition. Also, it might show an inclination to consider "conscientious beliefs" as those that are instilled in persons by God or religious authority. It is our opinion that the validity of a belief in terms of an orthodox tradition is not relevant. Rather, the sincerity of those who hold it and their ability to understand its consequences for their lives are the relevant issues in this sort of case. [EB: "Blood Transfusion," I, 289–293; Jonsen AR. Blood transfusions and Jehovah's Witnesses. *Critical Care Clinics* 1986; 2:91; *How Blood Can Save Your Life*. New York: Watch Tower Bible and Tract Society of New York, 1990.]

*RECOMMENDATION:* Mr. G.'s refusal should be respected. (a) If a Jehovah's Witness comes as a medical patient, as did Mr. G., the eventual possibility of the use of blood should be discussed and a clear agreement worked out between physician and patient about an acceptable manner of treatment. It should be learned whether the patient rejects autologous transfusion and dialysis as well as blood and blood products. Under no circumstances should the physician resort to deception. A physician who, in conscience, cannot accept being held to an inferior or dangerous standard of care should not enter into a patient-physician relationship or, if one already exists, should terminate it in the proper manner.

(b) If a Jehovah's Witness, who is known to be a confirmed believer, is in need of emergency care and refuses blood transfusion, the refusal ordinarily should be considered decisive. Even if the patient is mentally incapacitated at the time of the emergency, it can be presumed that the refusal represents the person's true wishes. However, if little is known about the patient and his or her status as a believer cannot be authenticated, treatment should be provided. In the face of uncertainty about personal preferences, it is our position that response to the patient's medical need should take ethical priority.

**2.5.2 P** Refusal of treatment by minor children who affirm unusual beliefs poses a particularly distressing problem for pediatricians.

**Case I.** James, a 14-year-old boy with acute lymphocytic leukemia, suffers his second relapse and fails to respond to chemotherapy. He is anemic and thrombocytopenic. He understands that transfusion would make him more comfortable, reduce the possibility of life-threatening bleeding, and perhaps allow him to leave the hospital. He affirms his belief as a Jehovah's Witness and refuses transfusion. His parents concur with his choice.

*COMMENT:* This boy is making an important decision: he is weighing his own discomfort against a belief about his eternal salvation. The medical value of the transfusion is, at best, limited. The boy is aware of his impending death and of the nature of his illness. He seems to show those characteristics of responsible decision-making that we require in adults, even if we might suspect that, if more mature, he would see his beliefs differently. It seems unethical to insist that he subordinate his beliefs for so transitory a benefit.

**Case II.** Karen, a 13-year-old, is sent from class to the school nurse complaining of severe headache and malaise. Noting her fever and irritability when moved, the nurse suspects meningitis. She calls the patient's mother, who says she will come directly to school. When the mother arrives, she informs the nurse that she and her husband are Christian Scientists. She says she will take

Karen home where a Christian Scientist practitioner will pray for her. Karen's father soon arrives and reinforces the mother's position. They ask the nurse not to call a physician. When the nurse warns them about the extreme seriousness of Karen's condition, they remind her that Christian Scientist practitioners are considered health professionals under the law of their state. When the nurse asks Karen whether she wishes to be seen by a doctor, she affirms that she, too, believes in the doctrines of Christian Science and declines.

*COMMENT:* The consequences of refusing medical treatment for meningitis are very serious. Even if this youngster were not disoriented due to her illness, it is dubious that she would appreciate the dire consequences. Also, Karen's illness, unlike James's, is sudden and unexpected, as well as curable. Legally, her parents' refusal can be viewed as neglect and subject to the sanctions of state law. [EB: "Alternative Therapies," I, 137–138.]

*RECOMMENDATION:* James's refusal of transfusions should be respected. Care should be directed to assuring his comfort. Karen's refusal of medical care should not be accepted and her parents' refusal opposed by providers, using the appropriate legal means. In general, the wishes of maturing children should be seriously considered in decisions about their care. Signs that the child has some comprehension of the situation and some appreciation of the consequences should be sought. Solicitous attention should be paid to helping them understand. The influences of fear and distress should be noted. Consultation with persons familiar with the psychology of the maturing child should be sought. Above all, nothing should be done to undermine the trust of the child in the adults who are responsible for care and upbringing.

## 2.5.3 Enigmatic Refusal

On occasion, refusal of care may appear enigmatic: it is difficult to discern why a person should refuse an obvious benefit or even difficult to know whether they are really refusing.

**Case.** At 2.2.2, Mr. Cure presented with signs and symptoms suggestive of bacterial meningitis. When he was told his diagnosis and told he would be admitted to the hospital for treatment with antibiotics, he refused further care, without giving a reason. The physician explained the extreme dangers of going untreated and the minimal risk of treatment. The young man persisted in his refusal. Other than this strange adamancy, he exhibited no evidence of mental derangement or altered mental status that would suggest decisional incapacity.

*COMMENT:* In this case the initial consent for diagnosis was implicit in the young man's presenting himself at the clinic. The patient's enigmatic refusal, however, unexpectedly introduced an incongruence between medical indications and patient preferences. It might be argued that the physician should simply permit the patient to refuse treatment and suffer the consequences, since the patient showed no objective signs of incapacitation or serious psychiatric impairment and since competent patients have the right to make their own (sometimes risky) decisions. However, where the risk of treatment is low and the benefit is great, the risk of nontreatment is high and the "benefits" of nontreatment are small, it is ethically obligatory for the physician to probe further to determine why the patient suddenly refused treatment. Despite the explanation given, has the patient somehow failed to understand and appreciate the nature of the condition or the benefits and risks of treatment and nontreatment? If patients understand the explanation, are they denying that they are ill? Or is the patient acting on the basis of some unexpressed fear, mistaken belief, or irrational desire? Through further discussion with the patient some of these questions might be answered. Assume, however, that after the most thorough investigation possible under the urgent circumstances there is no evidence that the patient fails to understand and nothing emerges to suggest denial, fear, mistake, or irrational belief. Should the patient's enigmatic refusal be respected? Since the medical condition is so serious, should treatment proceed even against the patient's will? This case poses a genuine ethical conflict between the patient's personal autonomy and the paternalistic values that favor medical intervention for the patient's own good. A clinical decision must be made quickly to treat or release the patient; good ethical reasons can be given for either alternative.

*RECOMMENDATION:* This patient's refusal is truly enigmatic. There is no evidence of incapacity to choose due to altered mental state (although the patient's high fever and brain infection might lead the physician to suspect some derangement). Further, there is no expression of an "unusual belief," for example, a religious objection to antibiotics. The patient simply refuses and will provide no reason for the refusal. Given both this enigmatic refusal and the urgent, serious need for treatment, the patient should be treated, even against his will, if this is possible. Should there be time, legal authorization should be sought. In offering this counsel, we reluctantly favor paternalistic intervention at the expense of personal autonomy. It is difficult to believe this young man wishes to die. The conscientious physician faces two evils: to honor a refusal that might not represent the patient's true preferences, thus leading to the patient's serious disability or death, or to override the refusal in the hope that, subsequently, the patient will recognize the benefit. This is a genuine moral dilemma: The principle of beneficence and the principle of autonomy seem to dictate contradictory courses of action. In medical care, dilemmas cannot merely be contemplated; they must be resolved. Thus, we resolve it in favor of treatment against the expressed preferences of this patient.

In this case, we accept as ethically permissible the unauthorized treatment of an apparently competent person. Recall that we endorsed Mr. Cope's refusal of a useful therapeutic procedure (2.5). How do these apparently inconsistent recommendations differ?

(a) The medical indications are significantly different. Mr. Cure has a critical disease, and low-risk antibiotic treatment will be effective in preventing serious harm. There is an opportunity for complete achievement of all medical goals. Mr. Cope is at risk of gangrene, but is not now critically ill.

(b) The consent situation is significantly different. In neither case is there behavioral evidence of psychiatric impairment, yet in both, the common psychological mechanism of denial may hinder good judgment. However, in the case of Mr. Cope, the refusal takes place after full disclosure of his problem, the proposed procedure and its risks. There has been an opportunity to discuss, persuade, and argue. In Mr. Cure's case, discussion is truncated. Efforts to discuss are rejected. Yet he has willingly come to be treated. There is strong suspicion that some crucial element of this negotiation is missing. It is this suspicion that leads the physicians, given the medical situation, to treat him against his wishes.

(c) In fact, something was missing. Mr. Cure's brother had nearly died twelve years ago of an anaphylactic reaction to penicillin. But while in the emergency department, Mr. Cure did not, and could not, recall this event and probing did not uncover it. Mention of antibiotics had triggered a psychological response of denial, which manifested itself in a refusal without reason. (Indeed, the patient did not recall these events when recovered.) The circumstances of his particular illness drew the physicians in the direction of rapid treatment. Even though they made an effort to uncover the source of the problem, they failed to do so, and urgent need for treatment took priority.

(d) The case illustrates that physicians are often pressured by circumstances to make decisions before all relevant information is known. Thus, the rightness or wrongness of the clinical decision always must be asserted in terms of what the clinician knows at the time of the decision. We include this complex and troubling case to illustrate how actual situations do, at times, yield ambiguous results. One can only strive to render decisions that are as fully and carefully analyzed as the circumstances permit.

### 2.5.4   Refusal of Information

Persons have a right to information about themselves. Similarly, they have the right to refuse information or to ask the physician not to inform them. Some patients may prefer not to have all the details spelled out for them and, once the options are explained, to allow the physician to decide. If this is clearly the patient's preference, it should be respected. On occasion, it will cause an ethical problem.

**Case.**   Mrs. Care, with MS, had shown little interest during the early years of her illness in learning about the possible course of her disease. She refused frequent offers by the physician to discuss it. However, on one of her repeated admissions for treatment of urinary tract infection, she states that, had she known what life would be like, she would have refused permission for treatment of other life-threatening problems. The patient's mental status is difficult to evaluate; some think she shows signs of early dementia. Should she have been informed of her prognosis at an earlier time even though unwilling to engage in such discussions with her physician?

*COMMENT:*   In this case, we are concerned with what the physician communicates and should communicate about diagnosis and, particularly, prognosis. Should the physician override the patient's stated preference not to know about her condition?

Should physicians withhold unpleasant information about prognosis to protect the patient from depression or other negative, potentially damaging emotions? Or should the patient be told enough to maximize her opportunity to plan her life in the face of future prospects? Although it is tempting to withhold information to protect the patient, a better alternative would be to give the patient general information sufficient to indicate the seriousness of her condition as well as the uncertainty about the time, the severity, and the extent of the problems that MS can cause. The middle ground avoids the extremes of withholding too much too long or disclosing too much too soon. Considerable tact is required to find the proper balance of disclosure and reticence. Furthermore, the disclosures made as the condition worsens must be adjusted in the light of the impairments to the patient's capacity. In some cases of late-stage MS an associated dementia appears. Thus, it would be advisable to make disclosures before the patient's capacity is so severely impaired that he cannot understand.

*RECOMMENDATION:*   Again we have a difficult case in which unpleasant but unavoidable moral choices must be made. Here we opt for more rather than less disclosure, especially because the condition, though untreatable, is long-lasting. Thus, the patient's long-term autonomy is respected more by providing as much information as possible to enable her to make more choices while she is physically and mentally able to learn coping mechanisms in advance. The short-term gains of ignorance are outweighed by the long-term benefits of knowledge.

**2.6**                        **ADVANCE PLANNING**

Persons are frequently concerned that when crucial decisions must be made about their medical care, they will no longer be capable of participating in those decisions. In recent years, the concept of advance planning has emerged and been widely promoted as a solution to that problem. The general term "advance planning" covers (a) the legal instrument entitled "Directive to Physicians" in the natural death acts enacted by various states; (b) the less formal "living will"; (c) the "durable power of attorney for health care."

Advance directives of some kind have explicit legal validity in nearly every state. Most people agree, at least in principle, with the idea that individuals should be permitted to express their preferences concerning termination of life-support in a legally effective document. In 1990, the United States Supreme Court stated that persons may have a constitutionally protected "liberty interest" in refusing unwanted medical treatment; this interest is not extinguished after mental capacity is lost. At the same time, the Court upheld a Missouri statute requiring "clear and convincing evidence" of an incapacitated person's prior wishes (Cruzan v. Missouri Dept. of Health, 1990). This implies the utility and legitimacy of advance directives. This reasoning comes after several decades in which the idea of advance directives has become both familiar and accepted in ethics and in law. Medicare regulations require hospitals to provide patients with information about their rights under local law to accept or refuse recommended care and to formulate advance directives. In the future, advance directives will become an increasingly important feature of routine medical care and especially important in terminal care. In light of these developments, physicians should become familiar with the provisions of advance directives that are legally valid in their locale. Physicians should know the differences between the three principal forms of advance directives: natural death acts, durable power of attorney for health care, and living wills.

Although the legality of advance planning has been formalized by legislation and upheld by courts, medical practice has been slow to respond to the preferences of terminally ill patients for less aggressive end-of-life care. Several empirical studies document that physicians are reluctant to discuss end-of-life issues with patients known to be dying. Physicians often failed to write DNAR orders for patients who had requested them to do so. Systematic attempts to improve communication, information, and conversation between patients and physicians met with little success. Nor did the use of outcome data or patient preferences influence physician practices. End-of-life care, at least in the intensive care setting, is currently driven more by traditional hospital and physician practices to prolong life than by patient preferences. [Support Principal Investigators. A controlled trial to improve care for seriously ill hospitalized patients. *JAMA* 1995; 274:1591–1598; EB: "Death and Dying, Advance Directives," I, 572–576; PBE: 131–132, 175–178; Advance Care Planning, Special Supplement, *Hastings Center Report* 1994; 24 (6); Haeckler C, Moseley R, Vawter D, eds. *Advance Directives in Medicine: Legal, Ethical and Medical Considerations.* New York: Praeger Press, 1989.]

### 2.6.1    Natural Death Acts

These are statutes passed by state legislatures. These statutes affirm a person's right to make decisions regarding terminal care and provide directions about how that right can be effected after the loss of decision-making capacity. Typically, they contain a model (or sometimes mandatory) document, called Directive to Physicians. These directives, which a patient can sign and give to the physician, typically are worded in this fashion: "If at any time I should have an incurable injury, disease, or illness certified to be a terminal condition by two physicians, and where the application of life-sustaining procedures would serve only to artificially prolong the moment of my death and where my physician determines that my death is imminent whether or not life-sustaining procedures are utilized, I direct that such procedures be withheld or withdrawn, and that I be permitted to die naturally." Various natural death acts contain specific provisions concerning a variety of topics, though the statutes vary in their coverage of them. The topics include personalized instructions, proxy appointments, whether a declaration is part of one's medical record, immunity clause for physicians who carry out patient directives, terminal condition diagnosis, witness requirements, permission or prohibition of withdrawing or withholding of ventilators, dialysis, artificial feeding and hydration, etc. Clinicians should know the specific features of the natural death acts of their states.

### 2.6.2    Living Wills

Advance directives may be communicated by a person to physicians, family, and friends in less formal, less legalistic fashion. Choice in Dying, a national organization that advocates expanded options for dying patients, provides a model document in which the operative words are "If I become unable, by reason of physical or mental incapacity, to make decisions about my medical care, let this document provide the guidance and authority needed to make any and all such decisions. If I am permanently unconscious or there is no reasonable expectation of my recovery from a seriously incapacitating or lethal illness or condition, I do not wish to be kept alive by artificial means."

"A Christian Affirmation of Life: A Statement on Terminal Illness," designed by the Catholic Health Association, contains the words, "I have a right to make my own decisions concerning treatment that might unduly prolong the dying process. If I become unable to make these decisions and have no reasonable expectation of recovery, then I request that no ethically extra-ordinary means be used to prolong my life but that my pain be alleviated if it becomes unbearable."

Other versions have been proposed. Individuals may choose to compose their own form of the living will. In some states, these personal documents are given legal standing equivalent to the natural death act's Directive to Physicians. Even if there is no explicit legal recognition of personal documents, physicians can and should respect and act upon them as expressions of their patient's preferences. [Choice in Dying. *A Good Death: Taking More Control at the End of Your Life*. Reading, Mass.: Addison-Wesley, 1992; *A Christian Affirmation of Life*. St. Louis: Catholic Hospital Association, 1974; Emanuel LL, Emanuel EJ. The medical directive: a new comprehensive advance care document. *JAMA* 1989; 261:3288.]

### 2.6.3   The Durable Power of Attorney for Health Care

This is a statute passed by a state legislature. It authorizes individuals to appoint another person, called an "attorney-in-fact" (who need not be an "attorney-at-law"), to act as their agent to make all health care decisions after they have become incapacitated. These statutes are particularly useful to physicians and hospitals because they authorize a specific decision-maker who presumably is familiar with the patient's wishes and values. These statutes give legal priority to the attorney-in-fact over all other parties, including next-of-kin. This clarifies the confusion that often exists about who in the family is the appropriate decision-maker for an incapacitated relative. This also avoids the bureaucratic burdens and costs of a legal proceeding to appoint a guardian or conservator.

### 2.6.4   The Patient Self-Determination Act

In 1990, Congress passed legislation requiring that all hospitals receiving federal funds, such as Medicare and Medicaid payments, must ask patients at the time of admission whether they have advance directives. If they do, patients are asked to submit copies for their records; if they do not, they are to be informed that they have the right to sign such a document and be given information about it. Although well intentioned, this legislation may not be helpful: the requirement is often casually fulfilled by an admitting clerk, information is skimpy and education almost nonexistent and the occasion often less than suitable. A hospital dedicated to patient self-determination would establish appropriate mechanisms for information and education and assure that patients' instructions are communicated to responsible parties.

## 2.6.5 Interpretation

Written advance directives are an important innovation in the expression of patient preferences. They allow persons to project their preferences into the future for consideration by those responsible for their care when they themselves are incapable of expressing preferences. Advance directives do, however, present some problems to those to whom they are addressed. As written documents, they employ terms that are vague, such as "if there is no reasonable expectation of recovery," or the direction to forgo "artificial means and heroic measures." Such language requires interpretation in the setting of the case. In addition, they sometimes do not specifically indicate which of the various means of life-sustaining treatments the patient would wish forgone. Thus, while these documents are helpful as evidence about the patient's prior preferences, they may not substitute for thoughtful and responsible interpretation in the particular case.

**Case I.** Mrs. Care, with MS, is now hospitalized due to aspiration pneumonia. She is alternatively obtunded and severely confused. She had given her physician a copy of the Directive to Physicians two years earlier. Now, in reviewing the directive, the physician notices the words (common in these documents), "the patient's death must be imminent, that is, death should be expected whether or not treatment is provided." Should the physician consider that if intubation is medically indicated, it should be withheld in accord with the patient's prior preferences?

**Case II.** A 70-year-old woman, very active and in good health, suffers a stroke after finishing a game of golf. She is admitted to the hospital unconscious and in respiratory distress. Studies show a brainstem and cerebellar infarct with significant edema involving the brainstem. She is provided ventilatory support. Her sister brings to the hospital a recently signed and witnessed "living will." It contains the words, "I fear death less than the indignity of dependence and deterioration." The patient is currently unable to communicate. She is intubated and has cardiac arrhythmias. The neurologist believes that this patient has a good chance of recovery with little functional deficit; he mentions to the sister that she might have some gait disturbance. The sister responds, "I know she wouldn't want to live with that." Should her physician, on becoming aware of the living will, extubate her? Should no-code orders be written?

**RECOMMENDATION:** In Case I, the physician may withhold intubation on the basis of the patient's advance directive. The words "whether or not treatment is provided" are a clumsy attempt to define the imminence of death. In this case, those words should not obstruct the fulfillment of the patient's preferences which, for one suffering from a deteriorating disease far advanced, seem quite clear. In Case II, withdrawing ventilatory support is premature given the facts of the case. It is as yet unclear whether this patient will suffer "the indignity of dependence and deterioration." However, if the patient's condition deteriorates, it may be appropriate to reconsider this opinion. At this point a DNAR order is also premature. However, if she recovers her ability to communicate and is competent, the exact meaning of her living will should be explored with her.

2.7                    **DECISION-MAKING FOR
THE MENTALLY INCAPACITATED PATIENT**

Persons receiving medical care are sometimes unable to make decisions in their own behalf. They can neither give consent to treatment nor refuse it. Their incapacity may arise from many causes. They may be unconscious and/or uncommunicative. They may be suffering from mental disabilities, either transitory, such as confusion or obtundation, or chronic, such as dementia or a psychopathology of some sort. When this occurs, decisions about the proper care of these persons must be made. The questions arise, who is the suitable decision-maker and what are the principles that should govern such decisions? [PBE: "A Framework of Standards for Surrogate Decisionmaking," 170–181, "Decision-making for Incompetent Patients," 241–249; Buchanan AE, Brock DW. *Deciding for Others: The Ethics of Surrogate Decision Making.* Cambridge: Cambridge University Press, 1989.]

### 2.7.1  Surrogate Decision-Makers

A person who is authorized to make a decision on behalf of another who is incapacitated is called a surrogate or a proxy. Traditionally, next of kin have been considered the natural surrogates, and medical providers have turned to family members for their consent. This practice appears to have been tacitly accepted in Anglo-American law, but until recently was rarely expressed in statutes. In recent years, many states have enacted legislation that gives specific authority to family members and ranks them in priority—e.g., spouse, parents, children, siblings. The durable power of attorney statutes also provide for a surrogate, the attorney-in-fact, who supersedes family members. These statutes avoid the need to seek judicial recourse, except in cases of conflict or doubt about legitimate decision-makers. Finally, all states have provisions for the judicial appointment of guardians or conservators for those declared judicially incompetent. [Areen J. The legal status of consent obtained from families of adult patients to withhold or withdraw treatment. *JAMA* 1987; 318:28.]

## 2.7.2 The Principle of Surrogacy

When someone other than a patient is granted authority to decide on behalf of the patient, that person's decisions must promote the patient's wishes and welfare. This is determined in two ways:

(a) If the patient has been able to express preferences in the past and has done so, the surrogate must use knowledge of these preferences, or at least of the known values of the individual, in making the decision. This is called "substituted judgment" and has been favored by many legal decisions (e.g., Quinlan, Saikewicz, Conroy, Spring, Brophy) (3.3.1).

(b) If the patient's own preferences are unknown or are unclear, the proxy must consider the "best interests" of the patient. This requires that the surrogate's decision promote the welfare of the individual; welfare is defined as those choices about relief of suffering, preservation or restoration of function, extent and quality of life sustained that reasonable persons in similar circumstances would be likely to choose (3.0.3).

## 2.7.3 Implied Consent

In life-threatening emergencies, patients may be unable to express their preferences or give their consent because they are unconscious or in shock. No surrogate may be available. In such situations, it has become customary for physicians to presume that the patient would give consent if able to do so, since the alternative would be death or severe disability. This is a reasonable presumption. The law has accepted it under the somewhat inaccurate title of "implied consent." This is a legal fiction, since the patient is not actually consenting: the physician is presuming. However, in law it provides the physician with a defense against a subsequent charge of battery (although it may not defend against charges of negligence if the emergency treatment falls below acceptable standards of care). From the ethical point of view, the principle of beneficence, which prescribes that there is a duty to assist someone in serious need of help, is the ethical justification for emergency treatment of the incapacitated person.

### 2.7.4    Statutory Authority to Treat

In all jurisdictions, statutes exist that authorize the physician to hold certain persons for psychiatric treatment against their will. These statutes pertain to persons who are suffering from mental disease, and the treatment authorized is treatment for mental disease. In addition, the person must be considered a danger to self or others. In some situations both mental disease and medical problems may be present. [EB: "Commitment to Mental Institutions," I, 418–423; ME: ch. 10, 305–307; McGarry L, Chodoff P. The ethics of involuntary hospitalization. In: Block S, Chodoff P, eds. *Psychiatric Ethics*. Oxford: Oxford University Press, 1981.]

**Case.**   A middle-aged man, known to the ER staff as psychotic and alcoholic, is brought to the hospital by a friend. He has been drinking, using heroin and is hallucinating that Viet Cong are attacking him. He is breathless, has fainted twice in the last hour, and is incontinent of urine. He says his heart is breaking through his chest. Still, he says he must leave the hospital because it is being bombed. The admitting resident writes in the chart, "I noted hallucinations and psychotic ideation; thus, I am putting the patient on a medical hold and keeping him in the hospital for observation. Diagnosis: paroxysmal supraventricular tachycardia. Medications: haloperidol, digitalis. Further evaluation: assess electrolytes."

*COMMENT:*   The question is whether the statutory authorization for involuntary hospitalization for psychiatric evaluation and treatment, sometimes called a "medical hold," allows medical treatment as well as treatment for mental illness. Each state's statute and local interpretations must be consulted for an answer. In general, the statutes seem to refer to mental illness alone as the justification for involuntary commitment and to its treatment as the sole permitted intervention. The question is probably not legally important if the treatment is lifesaving. In that case the legal doctrine of implied consent would suffice. If not lifesaving, but urgent and highly advisable, the physician is in a somewhat unclear situation. A clinical assessment of incapacity is made, but the patient has the legal right to refuse care unless declared incompetent. The physician should utilize the involuntary "hold" for psychiatric care and, if possible, seek authorization through hospital counsel to treat for medical problems as well.

### 2.7.5 P  Authority of Parents

Children, whose mental capacities mature with growth, are considered incompetent under the law. The medical care of infants and children is authorized by the usual surrogates, namely the parents of the child, or in unusual circumstances by other parties authorized by law. In addition, the law designates the age at which young persons are deemed capable of consent. Two ethical issues appear. First, it is sometimes necessary to determine the relevance and weight of parental preferences when these preferences conflict with the recommendations of providers. Second, children become capable of expressing their preferences at various ages. When they do express preferences, it is necessary to determine how reasonable and relevant these preferences are in matters of medical care.

Every child born has biological parents, but the authority of parents is a moral, social, and legal matter. It is commonly agreed that parents have the responsibility for the well-being of their children and that they have a wide range of discretion to determine in what that well-being will consist. At the same time, parental discretion is not absolute. Infants and children are, in this culture, considered persons, with certain interests and rights that must be acknowledged regardless of their parent's preferences. Thus, it is usually said that the best interests of the child set limits to the discretion of parents about the medical treatment of their offspring. Also, in this culture, the society as a whole has an interest in the welfare of children and accepts as an obligation the protection of children from harm, even at the hands of their parents. [Murray T. *The Worth of a Child*. Berkeley and Los Angeles: University of California Press, 1996.]

### 2.7.6 P  Determination of Parental Responsibility

In this society, biological parents may have various sorts of moral relationships to their offspring. Most parents eagerly and willingly accept their responsibility to nurture and educate their children. Some parents have conceived unwillingly and desire to be rid of their offspring before or immediately after birth. Others, due to various attitudes or pathologies, have no concern for the child they have borne. Other parties, such as adoptive parents, assume certain responsibilities, perhaps even before legally authorized. Due to shifting social relationships, various adults may undertake moral or legal care of the child at different times. Even if it is possible to determine who bears legal authority, it is not always easy to see who has moral responsibility. Thus, while biological and social parents are the natural surrogates for children, in certain circumstances they may be incapable or incompetent to carry out that responsibility.

### 2.7.7 P  Parental Incompetence

Pediatricians and other providers may occasionally suspect parents of serious incompetence in the care of their child. This suspicion must be cautiously evaluated. In some cases, a parent or parents may manifest the signs of a psychiatric disorder which might render them incapacitated for rational consideration of matters concerning their child. Indeed, a psychiatrically disabled parent may constitute a danger to the child. The existence and extent of psychiatric disease should be evaluated and, if indicated, legal steps taken to provide a surrogate decision-maker. Another sort of incompetence is manifested by parents who seem unable to comprehend the needs and interests of a child. Incompetence of this sort is most clearly manifest by overt and habitual physical abuse of a child. Failure to provide for the ordinary needs of a child may represent incompetence due to ignorance, moral turpitude, or substance addiction. In other cases, failure may be due to parental inexperience or to social conditions. Suspicion of incompetence should be evaluated for its degree, causes, remediability, and so forth. Most important, the alleged incompetence should be relevant to the problem at hand. Social workers and others expert at evaluation of social and environmental conditions are invaluable contributors. If suspicions are verified, legal remedies may be sought depending on the seriousness and urgency of the situation. Child protective services exist in every jurisdiction to assist, if this step is necessary.

### 2.7.8 P  Standard for Parental Preferences

When parents are properly identified and appear competent as decision-makers, they are morally and legally required to observe certain standards in their decision for their child. The federal Baby

Doe Rules state, "The decision to provide or withhold medically indicated treatment is, except in highly unusual circumstances, made by the parent or legal guardians. Parents are the decision-makers concerning care for their disabled infants, based on the advice and reasonable medical judgment of their physician . . . this role must be respected and supported unless they choose a course of action inconsistent with the standards established by law." (At 14880.) And, it may be added, inconsistent with moral principle. What standards, then, must guide parental choice?

(a) It is clear that medical inefficacy or futility justifies a parental decision to discontinue treatment. However, physicians and parents may disagree about the presence of these conditions. Parents may see as inefficacy the failure of a treatment to produce an immediate result or, overcome by the frustration of a long illness, conclude that treatment is futile. The physician has the duty to educate the parents, to explain the medical situation, and to strive to achieve a common understanding. Naturally, every effort must be made to reach an amicable understanding. However, it must be clear that the physicians and the institution have no ethical obligation to continue to provide treatment that, in their best professional judgment, is inefficacious or futile. In extreme cases, legal steps might be taken to relieve the institution of responsibility (1.4.1).

(b) It is equally true that physicians may be deluded by their own uncertainty, fear, or therapeutic or scientific zeal, and so fail to recognize or admit that current or proposed interventions are inefficacious or futile. This attitude, which can lead to ethical disasters, can be countered by rigorous honesty, genuine humility, and the willingness to listen to the opinions of others.

(c) Every pediatrician recognizes that the birth of a defective infant or the critical illness of a child can be a most traumatic experience for parents. Even the most lucid explanations of the medical problem can be misunderstood. It is difficult for parents to be properly informed and fully consenting surrogates. Nevertheless, it is also wrong to disqualify all parents as decision-makers on the supposition that no one can make good decisions in a crisis. Each case must be judged on its own. Serious efforts at psychologically and emotionally suitable communication must be made.

(d) If intervention is not clearly inefficacious or futile, decisions should be made in view of the best interests of the infant or child. The phrase "best interests" is explained at 2.7.2, 3.0.3, and 3.0.10 P. Here it should be noted that the interests of the decision-makers, namely, the parents and the physicians, or the interests of society at large are not the central focus: The interests of the patient constitute the standard for decisions made by others on behalf of that patient.

(e) A parental refusal of a recommended medical intervention should be respected unless the failure to provide the intervention would cause direct and serious harm to the child. Thus, a refusal to have a child immunized, while misguided, should be respected (unless it violates a statutory law), since it is impossible to demonstrate that an unimmunized child will be infected.

(f) In cases where there are differences of opinion between parents and physicians or between parents themselves, ethics committee review or ethics consultation may be helpful. If differences are irreconcilable, it may be necessary to have recourse to the legal system that has been established to protect the welfare of those incapable of protecting themselves. Such recourse is often extremely traumatic for all concerned, but it acknowledges that the infant or child, despite its inability to speak for itself, has a valued place in our society.

### 2.7.9 P  Parents with Unfamiliar Beliefs

Parents are granted wide discretion about the values they believe their children's lives should embody. The constitutional protection of religious liberty safeguards this discretion particularly strongly. Yet, as a matter of course, state law and local courts have commonly intervened to prevent parents from exposing children to serious risk of life and health on the basis of religious beliefs. Nevertheless, the child abuse laws of many states specifically declare that a child is not to be deemed abused merely because he or she is being treated for illness by spiritual means according to the tenets of a particular religion. Although often innocuous, these provisions sometimes put in peril the life or health of a child.

**Case I.**  An 11-year-old girl is brought to an ER from an automobile accident. She is unconscious, with shallow, gasping respirations and circumoral cyanosis. Severe contusions are noted across the chest, the left side of which moves paradoxically on inspiration. She is hypotensive and tachycardic. An intravenous infusion of Ringer's lactate is started. After intubation and stabilization of BP, a chest film confirms flail chest and possible intrathoracic hemorrhage. Insertion of a chest tube produced frank blood. As the child is being wheeled toward the operating room, the parents, who had arrived minutes before, step in front of the gurney and declare that they are Jehovah's Witnesses and refuse permission for blood transfusion.

**Case II.** In 2.5.2 P, we saw Karen, a 13-year-old girl, refusing medical attention for suspected meningitis and supported by her parents in this refusal on the grounds of Christian Science beliefs. We recommended that her parents' decision be challenged and legal steps be taken, if necessary. Suppose that this family lives in a state with a legal exemption for spiritual treatment of children.

**Case III.** Also in 2.5.2 P, James, a 14-year-old boy with acute lymphocytic leukemia refuses blood transfusions and is supported by his parents, who are Jehovah's Witnesses. We recommended that his refusal be respected.

*COMMENT:* Freedom of religion is highly valued and is protected by the Constitution of the United States. However, it is the freedom of the believer, capable of free and informed adherence to a faith, that is valued, not the effects of that belief on others, who do not or cannot accept it as their own. As Justice Holmes wrote, "Parents may make martyrs of themselves, but they are not free to make martyrs of their children" (Prince v. Massachusetts, 1944). It must be noted that neither of the two religious denominations mentioned above considers that their children will be damned by medical treatment, nor is there any evidence that they consider their children tainted or excluded from their community. Even in states with religious exemptions, physicians and hospitals should be prepared to bring before the Child Protective Agency and to the courts any case involving "medical interventions of clear efficacy that can prevent, ameliorate or cure serious disease, incapacity, or loss of life and interventions that will clearly result in prevention of future handicaps or disability for the child." [American Academy of Pediatrics Committee on Bioethics. Religious objections to medical care. *Pediatrics* 1997; 99:279.]

*RECOMMENDATION:* Blood transfusions should be initiated immediately in Case I. Court authority should be obtained only if delay will not jeopardize the child; otherwise, authority can be assumed on the basis of innumerable legal precedents allowing treatment in these conditions. In Case II, treatment should be started and authority sought to authorize such a decision. Every effort should be made to placate the parents and maintain good relations, but the child's well-being, not the parents, is the issue. Case III, however, is different in an important way: the boy is old enough to understand and to have some personal commitments and the prognosis is poor, even with treatment. Transfusion will not cure, but only palliate. It is ethical to omit transfusion in this case.

2.8                **THE LIMITS OF PATIENT PREFERENCES**

The preferences of patients have significant moral authority and must be taken into consideration in every treatment decision. Even the preferences of decisionally incapacitated patients are relevant to the decisions of those who must act in their behalf. However, the authority of patients' preferences is not unlimited. The ethical obligations of physicians are defined by the goals of medicine, as well as by the wishes of their patient. Physicians have no obligation to perform actions beyond or contradictory to the goals of medicine, even when requested to do so by patients. Thus, patients have no right to demand that physicians provide medical care that is contraindicated, such as unnecessary surgery, or treatments that are unorthodox, such as eccentric drug regimens. For example, even if state law permits persons to obtain and take laetrile for cancer or marijuana for pain or AIDS wasting, physicians are not obliged to comply with requests for these treatments, if they do not consider them appropriate medically or ethically. Similarly, if law eventually permits physicians to assist patients to commit suicide, individual physicians may decline to do so. Patients may not demand that physicians do anything illegal or unethical. For example, physicians must not provide certification of a disability that the patient does not have nor fail to report communicable diseases at the patient's request. Patients, or their authorized surrogates, may express a preference for continuing life-support by all available means, even when physicians judge that medical intervention is inefficacious or futile. Such a situation may raise intriguing and important conflicts between medical indications and patient preferences. [Brett AS, McCullough LB. When patients request specific interventions: defining the limits of the physician's obligation. *NEJM* 1986; 315:1347.]

**Case.** Mrs. H.W., an 87-year-old woman, is hospitalized after breaking her hip. She develops pneumonia and has a cardiopulmonary arrest. She is resuscitated and intubated, but has sustained severe anoxic encephalopathy. After six months, she is still respirator-dependent and is considered by neurology consultants to be in persistent vegetative state. Her husband is the authorized surrogate. He insists on continued support and presents a document entitled, "Expression of Intent to Caregivers," designed by the local medical society. This document authorizes withdrawal or withholding of interventions. It also contains the clause, "I want all measures to insure my survival (including hospitalization, consultations, surgery, life-support systems and tube feedings)." Mrs. H.W. had signed this document and checked that clause as her preference.

*COMMENT:* In this case, there is valid expression of patient preferences. Physicians judge that those preferences request continuance of procedures that are futile, provide no medical benefit, attain no goal of medicine and sustain a quality of life that is below minimal. However, Mrs. H.W. and her husband apparently consider continued organic life a value in itself and desire to sustain the quality of life currently possible. It is our opinion that patient preferences, important as they are, do not impose an obligation on physicians to act contrary to their best medical judgment. We have argued earlier that physicians are not obliged to prolong organic life when that is the only medical effect that intervention can achieve. We argue further that any requirement to employ medical skills contrary to medical and ethical judgment is equivalent to a kind of moral bondage. Physicians are neither mere technicians nor indentured servants, but autonomous professionals. The patient's values and preferences may be right and good in themselves; others have no obligation to further them against their best professional judgment. Physicians cannot undertake medical actions without the patient's permission, but may refrain from action that they consider unethical. Further, in cases where medical benefits are low or nonexistent and quality of life is below minimal, contextual factors, such as alternative use of resources, may be weighted more heavily (see Chapter 4).

*RECOMMENDATION:* In our opinion, the discontinuance of life-support contrary to the patient's and surrogate's wishes can be ethically justified. However, serious efforts should be made to win the surrogate's agreement. Negotiation might include the possibility of transfer to another institution. If these efforts fail, a court can be petitioned to issue an order clarifying legal rights and obligations. Hospitals are strongly advised to develop clear policies regarding cases such as these.

### 2.8.1 Conscientious Objection by Health Care Providers

Patients may express preferences that the physician finds morally objectionable. Traditionally, medical ethics has required physicians to abstain from moral judgments about their patients in regard to medical care. *Examples:* An ER physician is expected to provide competent care to the wounded assailant of an elderly person as well as to the assaulted party; a physician should treat, without censure, venereal disease contracted in what the physician considers an immoral liaison.

However, physicians and nurses have their own personal moral values. On occasion, they may be asked not merely to tolerate what they consider immorality but to participate in effecting an immoral action desired by the patient. *Examples:* A male patient requests a physician who considers transsexualism morally wrong to prescribe female estrogens in order to promote secondary female characteristics; a Catholic nurse is asked to participate in an abortion.

Physicians and nurses may refuse to cooperate in actions they judge immoral on grounds of conscience. It is important, in forming one's conscience, to separate the moral values to which one is committed from personal distaste or prejudice. *Example:* A physician refuses to undertake the care of a Jehovah's Witness with a hemorrhagic diathesis "on moral grounds," while in fact the physician does not like to feel impotent or run the risk of "losing a patient." Institutions and programs should establish policy about conscientious objection and make the policy clear to those who work in that institution or program. [PBE: "Conscientious Objection," 497–483; Childress J. Civil disobedience, conscientious objection and evasive non-compliance: a framework for the analysis and assessment of illegal actions in health care. *J Med Philos* 1985; 10:73.]

### 2.9 FAILURE TO COOPERATE WITH MEDICAL RECOMMENDATIONS

Physicians have the responsibility to recommend to patients a course of treatment or other behavior that would, in the physician's best judgment, help the patient. Patients have the right to be informed of the benefits and risks associated with these recommendations and to accept them or refuse them. These rights and responsibilities are in principle quite clear. However, patients may accept the recommendations of physicians and fail to act on them, yet continue to seek the care of the physician. This is the problem known as "noncompliance" (a term that many dislike due to its paternalistic overtones). We prefer to use the expression, "failure to cooperate with medical recommendations." The problem posed to the physician is how to carry out his or her ethical responsibilities to a patient who asks for help but for some reason does not, or cannot, avail himself or herself of what is offered.

**Case.** Mr. Cope, a 42-year-old man with insulin-dependent diabetes, was first diagnosed at age 21. He complied with an insulin and dietary regimen quite faithfully. He nevertheless experienced frequent episodes of ketoacidosis and hypoglycemia, which necessitated repeated hospitalizations and emergency room care. For the past few years, his diabetes has been better controlled, and he required hospitalization only once for ketoacidosis associated with acute pyelonephritis. He has been actively involved in his diabetic program. He has been scrupulous about eating habits and maintained an ideal body weight. He is knowledgeable about the use of insulin and currently takes 30 units neutral protein Hagedorn insulin (NPH), 10 units regular insulin each morning and 15 units NPH in the evening. On this program, his urine fractionals are negative, his fasting blood sugars are less than 100 mg/dl and his two-hour postprandial sugars are usually below 140 mg/dl. Twenty-one years after the onset of diabetes, he appears to have no functional impairment from his disease. Funduscopic examination reveals some neovascularization, which was treated with laser therapy, and urinalysis shows persistent proteinuria (less than 1 g/day). He has no neurological or gastrointestinal symptoms.

However, after a stormy divorce and loss of an executive position, the patient has changed in several ways. In the three years following divorce, he has gained 60 pounds and has become negligent about his insulin medication. He has also started to abuse alcohol excessively and had a serious automobile accident while driving under the influence. During these years, he has required frequent admissions to the hospital for diabetic complications including (1) ketoacidosis, (2) traumatic and poorly healing foot ulcers, and (3) alcohol-related problems. While in the hospital, his diabetes is easier to manage, but even while in the hospital he is frequently found in the cafeteria eating excessively. On two admissions, blood alcohol levels in excess of 200 mg/dl were detected. Soon after discharge from the hospital, his diabetic control lapses.

His physician is frustrated. He blames the recurring medical problems on the patient's unwillingness to participate actively in his own care. The physician tells him he could easily control his diabetic problem by merely resuming health habits he had pursued for so many years, that is, by losing weight, by taking his insulin regularly, and by drinking alcohol in moderation. The patient asserts that he will change his life-style but on discharge from the hospital he relapses almost immediately. The physician urges him to seek psychiatric consultation. He agrees. The psychiatrist suggests a behavior modification program, which proves unsuccessful. Finally, aversion therapy is suggested. His physician hesitates to advise him to participate in this program.

Mr. Cope continues to require hospitalization lasting 7 to 10 days every month or two. After 10 years of working closely with this patient, the physician considers withdrawing from the therapeutic relationship because he senses he is no longer able to help the patient. "Why keep this up?" he said. "It's useless. Whatever I do, he undoes." The patient resists this suggestion. He complains the physician is punishing his drinking by abandoning him. Is persistent failure to comply with medical advice relevant to an ethical decision to withdraw from a case?

*COMMENT:*    (a) Patients such as Mr. Cope are very frustrating to those who attempt to care for them. Occasionally the physician will accuse the patient (in words or in attitude) of being irresponsible. The patient engages constantly and apparently willfully in behavior that poses serious risk to health and even to life. Such patients place great strain on the doctor-patient relationship; often the accommodation between doctor and patient founders because of the strain.

(b) The accusation of irresponsibility can be an example of the ethical fallacy of "blaming the victim"; the actual fault may lie with a more powerful party who finds a way to lay the blame for his own failure on the ones who suffer its effects. The poor, for example, were accused of lack of ambition by industrialists who paid paltry wages for difficult work. Similarly, the apparent irresponsibility of patients may be an impression created by the failure of a physician to educate, support, and convey personal concern and interest in the patient. It may be more than an impression: persons may be rendered incapable of caring responsibly for themselves by the way their physician deals with them. An excessive paternalism may stifle responsibility, while the physician's lack of personal concern may encourage tendencies to neglect medical advice. While Mr. Cope's physician did not have these faults and, indeed, had made solicitous efforts to support Mr. Cope, the problem may lie behind many cases of failure to cooperate.

*RECOMMENDATION:* (a) It is important to determine whether and to what extent the patient is acting voluntarily or involuntarily. Much uncooperative behavior is voluntary in the sense that the patient demonstrates no signs of pathological behavior. Patients either choose to ignore the regimen in favor of other behaviors they value more than health (a goal that, in an asymptomatic disease, may not seem very urgent or immediate) or fail to cooperate because of such factors as irregular routine, complicated regimen, habitual forgetfulness, or poor explanation by the physician. Some noncompliance arises from profound emotional disturbance and ambivalence.

(b) If the physician judges that noncooperation arises from the patient's persistence in voluntary health risks, reasonable efforts at rational persuasion should be undertaken. If these fail, it is ethically permissible for the physician to adjust therapeutic goals and do the best in the circumstance; it is also ethically permissible to withdraw from the case, after advising the patient how to obtain care from other sources.

(c) If contextual features, such as inability to pay for medicines, inadequate housing, etc., are at the source of noncooperation, help should be provided to improve these circumstances. A large literature, often unfamiliar to physicians, suggests many helpful stratagems to correct obstacles of this sort. [Haynes RB, Taylor DW, Sackett DL. *Compliance in Health Care.* Baltimore: Johns Hopkins University Press, 1979.]

(d) If noncooperation arises from psychological pathology, the physician has a strong ethical obligation to remain with the patient, adjusting treatment plans to the undesirable situation. Professional assistance in treating the pathology should be sought. The physician will experience great frustration, but the frustration is not, in itself, sufficient to justify leaving the patient. Additional circumstances, however, may contribute to a justification.

### 2.9.1 The Problem Patient: Noncritical

Failure to cooperate with medical recommendations occurs in situations where the results, while harmful to the health of the patient, are not critical.

**Case.** Mr. Cope was admitted for inpatient treatment of obesity with a protein-sparing modified fasting regimen. He was found repeatedly in the cafeteria cheating on the diet. His physician made reasonable efforts to persuade him to change his behavior.

*COUNSEL:* It would be ethically permissible for the physician to abandon therapeutic goals and to discharge the patient from the hospital. These goals are unachievable because of the patient's failure to participate in the treatment program.

### 2.9.2 The Problem Patient: Critically Ill

Is it ever justifiable to discharge a "problem patient" who has a critical illness requiring in-hospital treatment? Just as we believe that noncritically ill patients can be discharged if they repeatedly frustrate physicians' efforts to provide needed medical assistance, we also believe that noncooperation that directly counters the physician's effort can justify discharging a patient who is critically ill and in need of care. The situation, however, is more serious and requires added considerations before a decisive conclusion can be reached.

**Case.** R.A., an intravenous drug addict, is admitted for the third time in three years with a diagnosis of infective endocarditis. Three years before, he required mitral valve replacement for *Pseudomonas* endocarditis, and one year ago he required replacement of the prosthetic valve after he developed *Staph aureus* endocarditis. He now presents again with *Staph aureus* endocarditis of the prosthetic valve.

After one week of antibiotic therapy, he continues to have positive blood cultures. He consents to open heart surgery to replace again the infected prosthetic mitral valve. For 10 days postoperatively (four in the intensive care unit) he is cooperative with his management and antibiotic treatment. On this treatment he becomes afebrile, and blood cultures are negative.

He then begins to behave erratically. He leaves his room and stays away for hours, often missing his medications. On several occasions a urine screening test demonstrates the presence of opiates and quinine, suggesting that he is using illicit narcotics even while being treated for infective endocarditis. On two separate occasions he punches nurses who scold him for being away from his room. On the eleventh postoperative day he is discovered by hospital security guards in his bathroom selling injectable narcotics to another patient. His roommate in the hospital had observed these dealings for several days, but the patient threatened to kill the roommate if he told anyone about these transactions. When all this information becomes known to the patient's physician, the patient is asked to leave the hospital immediately. Despite the fact that the patient's infective endocarditis has not been treated optimally, he was discharged from the hospital against his will.

*COMMENT:* Considerations leading to an ethical justification of this decision are:

(a) The patient's use of intravenous street drugs at the same time that his physicians were attempting to eradicate his infective endocarditis indicated that the likelihood of medical success in this case, both short-term and long-term, was not great. Physicians are not obliged to treat people who persist in actions that run directly counter to the goals of such treatment.

(b) The patient wanted to be treated and, at the same time, continued his abusive and illegal behavior. The physicians are obliged to determine that the patient has the mental capacity to make such choices and that he was not suffering from a metabolic encephalopathy (2.2). On the other hand, the physicians are not obliged to deal with the patient's long-standing sociopathic behavior pattern.

(c) This patient's physicians (who were hospital-based) had obligations both to this patient and to their other hospitalized patients. This patient's behavior of selling narcotics to other inpatients and of terrorizing his roommate compromised the care other patients of the same physician were receiving. This patient, then, posed a direct and serious threat to other identifiable persons.

*RECOMMENDATION:* Mr. R.A. is truly a difficult patient. Providers should make a sympathetic effort to understand the complex causes of his behavior and motivations. They should avoid "blaming the victim." Serious efforts should be made to counsel, to negotiate and to develop "contracts" that make clear to him the consequences of his behavior. Early and repeated warnings should be issued. One identified provider should be responsible for dealing with this patient. In the end, if all fails, it is ethical to dismiss him from treatment. Providers of last resort, such as county hospitals, may follow this advice, although their efforts to remedy the situation may have to be more intense. Obviously, legal advice should be sought.

### 2.9.3   The Problem Patient: Socially Unacceptable

Our reasoning in the above case does not apply to most patients who present with critical illness, even those illnesses for which the patient might be held responsible.

**Case.**   A 35-year-old chronic alcoholic with a long criminal record had emergency portacaval shunt for variceal bleeding. He continued to drink alcohol. Two years later, he presented within three months with acute bleeding from esophageal varices.

*COMMENT:*   The problem with this patient is twofold. First, there is the suspicion that he will appear again, in the near future, with the same problem. Second, his problem was caused by personal behavior that is socially unacceptable. The first problem raises the issues in Chapter 4 about allocation of scarce resources (4.4); when the patient does become a repeater, the considerations mentioned there are relevant to a decision about his treatment. The second problem is discussed under Quality of Life (3.0.8). It should be noted that some harmful personal habits are commonly considered more socially unacceptable than others. Substance abuse is strongly disapproved, while overeating, fast driving, not wearing seatbelts, or engaging in dangerous sports are tolerated or even praised. Many conditions requiring expensive medical treatment are caused by behaviors that are socially accepted. Thus, singling out socially disapproved behaviors as less deserving of treatment reflects social prejudices rather than logic.

*RECOMMENDATION:*   This patient should be managed with aggressive medical and surgical means in an effort to control his hemorrhage and to reverse his blood loss. It takes more than past behavior to warrant physicians' withdrawing from the treatment of serious illness; indeed, the patient's past history should be ignored in most cases except insofar as it is medically relevant. Rather, refusal to treat a patient can be ethically justified in view of a person's behavior in the present circumstances only when that behavior makes achievement of medical goals impossible.

### 2.9.4 Signing Out Against Medical Advice

Mr. R.A., the patient described in 2.9.2, might leave the hospital before physicians judge his treatment adequate. When patients choose to discharge themselves in this manner, most hospitals request them to sign a statement confirming that they are leaving against medical advice (AMA). Of course, the patients cannot be forced to sign the statements; they have the right to leave at will. The document merely provides legal evidence that the patient's departure was voluntary and that the patient was warned by the physician about the risks of leaving. This warning, carried out as patiently and carefully as possible, is the ethical duty of the physician.

### 2.9.5 Withdrawing from the Case

At times, such as in the case of Mr. Cope, the physician may serve the patient best by deciding to dissolve the physician-patient relationship and by helping the patient to find another physician. The physician's principal goal is to help patients in the care of their health. If, for whatever reasons, this proves impossible, the physician may best demonstrate ethical responsibility by withdrawing from the case and finding another physician who might be more successful with the patient in these particular circumstances.

### 2.9.6 Abandonment

Physicians who terminate the relationship with a patient sometimes wonder whether they can be charged with "abandonment." The legal charge of abandonment can arise when the physician, without giving timely notice, ceases to provide care for a patient who is still in need of medical attention or when the physician is dilatory and careless (e.g., failure to visit the patient in the hospital or failure to judge the patient's condition serious enough to warrant attention). A charge of abandonment can usually be countered by showing that the patient did receive warning in sufficient time to arrange for medical care. There is no legal obligation on the physician to arrange for further care from another physician, although there is a legal obligation to provide full medical records to the new attending physician. If the physician does intend to maintain the relationship with the patient but will be unavailable for a time, there is a legal obligation to arrange for coverage by another physician. Failure to do so can be construed as abandonment. [Holder AR. *Medical Malpractice Law*. New York: John Wiley, 1975, ch. 12.]

Thus, a physician may withdraw from the care of a patient without legal risk. Still, a decision to do so should meet ethical as well as legal standards. Physicians inherit an ethical tradition that calls upon them to undertake difficult tasks and even risks for the care of persons in need of medical attention. Inconvenience, provocation or dislike are not sufficient reasons to exempt a physician from that duty. That obligation is, of course, limited by several conditions. If the patient absorbs excessive time and energy, drawing the physician away from other patients, if the patient is acting in ways to frustrate the attainable medical goals, or if the patient is endangering others by overt action, the ethical obligation to continue to care would be diminished. These conditions appear to be verified in the case of Mr. R.A.

## 2.10                          ALTERNATIVE MEDICINE

Many persons seek care from providers who are not trained in conventional scientific medicine. These providers, some of whom are licensed in their own forms of health care, apply physical, psychological, and herbal remedies that are not commonly recognized as scientific or proven as effective by clinical trials. The most common of these providers are naturopaths, homeopaths, chiropractors, and acupuncturists. Methods include spiritual healing, physical manipulation, special diet, imaging, relaxation techniques, massage, and vitamin therapy. These methods are described as "alternative" or "complementary" medicine. Often patients who are under the care of regular practitioners are also seeking care from these alternative practitioners. What is the obligation of the physician toward such patients? [EB: "Alternative Therapies," I, 135–143; Eisenberg DM, Kessler RC, Foster C, Norlock FE, Calkins DR, Delbanco TL. Unconventional medicine in the United States. Prevalence, costs and patterns of use. *NEJM* 1993; 328:246–252; Ernst E. The ethics of complementary medicine. *J Med Ethics* 1996; 22: 197–198.]

**Case.** A 64-year-old man has been under the care of a family physician for increasingly severe osteoarthritis. On one visit, he complains of dizzy spells. Workup reveals no specific cause for his dizziness. In discussing his arthritis, he tells his doctor that he gets some relief from mushroom tea. The physician has seen reports of illness due to "kombucha tea," which, although called "mushroom tea," is actually a colony of bacteria and yeast fermented in sweetened tea. The physician inquires and the patient reluctantly admits that he has been seeing a "natural healer" who sold him the concoction. [McNaughton C, Eidsness LM. Ethics of alternative therapies. *South Dakota J Med* 1995; 48:209–211.]

*COMMENT:* The large number of persons who visit alternative practitioners (estimated to be about one of every three adult Americans, making some 425 million visits yearly—more than are made to regular primary care practitioners) commonly do so in conjunction with care from regular practitioners, using unconventional therapies as adjuncts rather than replacements of conventional therapy. The majority of these patients do not inform their regular physician about their use of alternative treatment. Preferences for alternative treatments are often motivated because they are less arduous and less costly than conventional treatments, or because patients are frustrated with the failure of conventional treatment to assuage problems such as chronic back pain, headache, insomnia, anxiety and depression. Most conventional practitioners know little about alternative medicine, and most commonly disdain it and disparage its claims.

*RECOMMENDATION:* (a) Regular physicians should encourage their patients to reveal their use of alternative medications; disparaging remarks inhibit patients from speaking about what they fear will lead to anger or ridicule on the physician's part.

(b) Regular physicians should try to attain a better understanding of the healing systems to which patients have frequent recourse and to appreciate their beneficial features.

(c) When patients are using alternative therapies for serious conditions to the neglect of demonstrated efficacious therapies, or when they are utilizing therapies that have toxic effects, physicians should carefully explain the consequences of such a course, realizing that a clumsy approach may be more likely to confirm the patient in the use of inadvisable therapy than to convert them to the physician's recommended ones.

(d) In serious conditions, where the use of alternative medicine may impede cure or be dangerous, the physician should ask the patient's permission to contact the alternative provider, explain the situation, and attempt to work out a program that will be acceptable to the patient and conformable to the ethics of the providers.

(e) Hospitals should develop policies that acknowledge the prevalence of alternative therapies and establish guidelines for acceptable collaboration.

**2.11**                            **SUMMARY**

The preferences of patients demand respect on the basis of the ethical principle of autonomy. Respect entails that patients should be truthfully provided the information necessary for an informed consent or refusal of treatment. Their preferences should be followed, although certain exceptions, based on ethical principles other than respect for autonomy, are allowed. Special provisions for decisionally incapacitated patients should accord with the principles of ethics as well as with the law of local jurisdictions. Standards for surrogacy should be observed and the prior expressed wishes of patients should be honored, to the extent possible. The principle of autonomy should be seen as vital to ethical practice and to ethical clinical decisions, although other moral principles may on occasion limit its observation.

# CHAPTER 3

# Quality of Life

**3.0**   Quality of life is the third topic that must be reviewed in order to define and resolve a problem in clinical ethics. Analysis of a clinical case, after reviewing medical indications and patient preferences, should proceed to a discussion of the patient's quality of life prior to the current illness and expected quality of life with or without treatment. This chapter is devoted to explaining the difficult notion of quality of life, its implications for clinical decisions, and to suggesting certain distinctions and cautions that should be observed in discussing the notion in the context of clinical care.

The most fundamental goal of medical care is the improvement of the quality of life of those who need and seek care. All of the more particular goals stated in 1.1, such as relief of pain and restoration of function, are aspects of this fundamental one. Patients seek medical attention because they are distressed by symptoms, worried by doubts about their health, or disabled by accidents and disease. The physician responds by diagnosing, treating, curing, comforting, and educating. These activities aim at improvement of the quality of the patient's life.

In many clinical situations, that improvement can be effected easily and rapidly: Mr. Cure's headache, stiff neck, and malaise can be relieved by administering an antibiotic that will eliminate the infection causing them. The quality of his life, impaired by the infection, is rapidly restored to normal. In other situations, the quality of the patient's life is seriously disrupted by a disease for which no cure is available; the patient will become progressively disabled. Medical intervention aims at reduction of discomfort and maintenance of functions to the extent possible: Mrs. Care's quality of life is generally diminished but made "tolerable" by various medical, nursing, and rehabilitative interventions. In other situations, a patient's disease may be treated by an intervention that may cure the disease or retard its progress but, at the same time, reduce the quality of the patient's life. For example, Mr. Cope, a patient with brittle diabetes, will have to endure a strict dietary and insulin regimen; Ms. Comfort underwent a mastectomy and multiple courses of chemotherapy and radiotherapy in the attempt to conquer her cancer.

The evaluation of quality of life enters into all discussions about appropriate medical care. Physicians and patients must determine what level of quality is desirable, how it is to be attained, and at what risks and disadvantages. Unlike the risks and benefits considered in medical interventions, which are relatively immediate, quality-of-life considerations focus on the long-term consequences of accepting or refusing a recommendation for medical intervention. These considerations should be a part of all serious discussion of medical choices; however, they raise ethical questions in several ways: (1) when there is a notable divergence between quality of life as assessed by physicians and by patients; (2) when patients are unable to express their evaluation of the quality of life they wish to have; (3) when quality of life is used as an objective standard for rationing of care. The first two issues are discussed in this chapter; the third is discussed in Chapter 4. [EB: "Life, Quality of Life in Clinical Decisions," III 1352–1358, "Life, Quality of Life in Legal Perspective," III 1361–1366; PBE: "The Centrality of Quality of Life Judgments," 215–219, "The Value and Quality of Life," 305–313.]

### 3.0.1 Meaning of Quality of Life

Despite the importance of the notion of quality of life in clinical medicine, the phrase is not easy to define. It is, as one judicial opinion stated, "vague and perhaps ill-chosen" (Saikewicz, 3.3.1). In general, the phrase expresses a value judgment: the experience of living, as a whole or in some aspect, is judged to be "good" or "bad," "better" or "worse." In recent years, efforts have been made to develop measures of quality of life that can be used to evaluate outcomes of clinical interventions. Such measures list a variety of physical functions, such as mobility, performance of activities of daily living, absence or presence of pain, social interaction, and mental acuity. Scales are devised to rate the range of performance and satisfaction with these aspects of living. Many of these assessments are disease-specific but one, called QALY (Quality Adjusted Life Years), attempts to provide a global measurement based upon the ratio between states of health and life expectancy. These various measures aim to provide an objective description of what is inevitably a highly subjective and personal evaluation. In this sense, quality of life is more relevant to policy than to clinical decisions. Even when measures are based on empirical surveys of what persons consider valuable, individuals may depart, often in striking ways, from the general view. The empirical studies themselves are difficult to design and limited in application.

Quality-of-life judgments, then, are not based on a single dimension, nor are they entirely subjective or objective. They must take into account personal and social function and performance, symptoms, prognosis, and the subjective values that patients ascribe to quality-of-life considerations. Several important questions must be raised: (a) Who is making the evaluation—the person living the life or an observer? (b) What criteria are being used to evaluate? Finally, the crucial ethical question: (c) What sorts of clinical decisions, if any, are justified by reference to quality-of-life judgments? The answer to this question is relevant to discussions about forgoing life-sustaining measures as well as to allocation of resources. [EB: "Economic Concepts in Health Care," II, 641–657; "Health-Care Resources, Allocation of," II, 1067–1084; McDowell I, Newell C. *Measuring Health. A Guide to Rating Scales and Questionnaires.* New York: Oxford University Press, 1996; Spilker B, ed. *Quality of Life Assessments in Clinical Trials.* New York: Raven Press, 1990; Menzel PT. *Strong Medicine: The Ethical Rationing of Health Care.* New York: Oxford University Press, 1990.]

### 3.0.2 Sanctity of Life and Quality of Life

This distinction is sometimes used to describe differing attitudes toward protection of human life. Proponents of sanctity of life will insist that diminished quality of life never justifies abandoning life-sustaining treatment. Sanctity of life is sometimes associated with the idea that human life is so valuable that it must be preserved at all costs, under any conditions, for as long as possible. This view is sometimes called vitalism and can be rooted in either religious or secular beliefs. Although vitalistic beliefs may not be explicit in medicine, much of medical practice draws its energy from vitalism. The desire to preserve organic life even when all other human functions are irreparably lost reflects a vitalistic attitude. The meaning of sanctity of life and its use as an ethical argument can be reviewed in the philosophical or theological literature. [Clouser D. The sanctity of life: an analysis of a concept. *Ann Intern Med* 1973; 78:119; McCormick R. The quality of life, the sanctity of life. *Hastings Center Report* 1978; 8:32; Rosner F. *Modern Medicine and Jewish Ethics.* New York: Yeshiva Press, 1986.]

### 3.0.3   Distinctions

It is important to distinguish between two uses of the phrase "quality of life." Failure to do so can cause confusion in clinical discussions.

(a) The personal satisfaction expressed or experienced by an individual in his or her physical, mental, and social situation. We call this "personal evaluation."

*EXAMPLE I:*   A 23-year-old gymnastics instructor who is paralyzed due to a cervical spinal cord lesion may say, "My life isn't as bad as it looks: I've come to terms with my loss and discovered the powers of the mind."

*EXAMPLE II:*   A 68-year-old artist who is a chronic diabetic now faces blindness and multiple amputations. She says: "I wonder if I can endure a life of such poor quality?"

(b) The evaluation of an onlooker of another's experiences of personal life. We call this "observer evaluation."

*EXAMPLE I:*   A parent says of a 29-year-old retarded son with an IQ of 40, "He used to seem so happy, but now he's become so restless and difficult—what kind of quality of life does he have?"

*EXAMPLE II:*   An 83-year-old woman with advanced senile dementia, who is bedridden and tube-fed is described by the nurses as "having poor quality of life."

*COMMENT:*   Reference to quality of life in a clinical discussion is natural and necessary, but because the phrase can be used in so many ways, its invocation can cause confusion. Distinctions must be made.

(a) The judgment of poor quality of life may be made by the one who lives the life or by an observer. It often happens that lives which observers consider of poor quality are lived quite satisfactorily by the one living that life. Human beings are amazingly adaptive. They can make the best of the options available. For example, the quadriplegic gymnastics instructor may be a person of extraordinary motivation; the blind artist may enjoy a vivid imagination; the retarded person may experience simple pleasures. Thus, if patients can evaluate and express their own quality of life, other parties should not presume to judge but seek the patients' opinions. Similarly, when the person's own evaluation is not or cannot be known to others, those others should be extremely cautious in applying their own values.

(b) Poor quality of life might mean, in general, that the sufferer's experiences fall below some standard that the speaker considers desirable. But in each case the experience in question is different; it may be pain, loss of mobility, presence of multiple debilitating health problems, loss of mental capacity and of the enjoyment of human interaction, loss of joy in life, and so on. Poor quality of life, then, refers to many quite different circumstances.

(c) Evaluation of the quality of life, like life itself, changes over time. The artist's concern may arise from a temporary depression that will resolve as she discovers her future possibilities; the gymnastics instructor may later become deeply depressed. Thus, providers of care must take care not to make momentous decisions on the basis of possibly transitory conditions.

(d) The evaluation may reflect bias and prejudice. When sufferers from mental retardation are said to have "poor quality of life," this may reflect our cultural bias in favor of intelligence and productivity. Prejudice may incline some to judge that persons of such a race, social status or sexual preference cannot possibly live "good quality" of life.

(e) The evaluation may reflect socioeconomic conditions rather than the experienced life of the patient, for example, the lack of home care, of rehabilitation, or special education. These obstacles, while very real, can often be overcome by planning and effort on the part of providers.

*EXAMPLE:*   Dax Cowart, described in the Introduction, believed at first that his disabilities caused by the explosion—blindness, disfigurement, crippling—would make his life intolerable and not worth living. He wanted to refuse treatment and be allowed to die. His personal assessment of his quality of life was that it was too low to go on living. Later Dax revised his earlier assessment as he gradually learned to use his mind more effectively, to enjoy simple pleasures, and to cope with his frustrations. He became a lecturer about his own story and an advocate for the rights of patients and the disabled. He graduated from law school, passed the bar, and is practicing law. He continues to deal daily with frustrations of his disabilities, but has achieved a quality of life that he could not previously imagine. Many students, on viewing the videotape *Please Let Me Die,* where Dax is shown at a time of extreme distress and deficits, judge his life to be of such poor quality that it could not be worth living. He would have agreed at that time; he now views his life differently (although he still believes that he should not have been deprived of the right to end his life). In addition to Dax's personal assessment, those who provided care for him— physicians, surgeons, and nurses—offered observer assessments that were more optimistic than Dax's. They had seen patients equally badly burned recover to an acceptable quality of life and tended to impose this experience on Dax. This example reminds us of the need for caution in applying quality-of-life judgments in clinical decisions.

### 3.0.3   Best Interest Standard and Quality of Life

At 2.7.2, we noted that authorized persons, such as next of kin, guardians or parties holding durable powers of attorney, in making decisions for the patient, are required to follow previous known wishes of the patient or, if their wishes are not known, to act in their best interests. The notion of "best interest," drawn from legal parlance, is often difficult to apply to health care situations. In general, it refers to the quality of life that a "reasonable person" would choose were he or she able to do so. "Reasonable person" is a useful fiction, devised to express what we might expect the priorities of most human beings to be in a typical situation. This is quite vague. Two steps can dispel some of this vagueness. First, what counts as an interest should be designated, as much as possible, from the viewpoint of the one for whom the judgment is being made. The interests common to competent, intelligent persons may not even occur to persons who suffer significant limitations of these faculties. Still, they have interests in the pursuit and securing of certain values suited to their limitations. The proxy decision-makers should attempt to view the world of such persons through their eyes. Second, the interests at stake should be judged by reference to more objective, societally shared values, rather than more individualized values. In the words of the President's Commission:

> In assessing whether a procedure or course of treatment would be in a patient's best interest, the surrogate must take into account such factors as the relief of suffering, the preservation or restoration of functioning, and the quality as well as the extent of life sustained. An accurate assessment will encompass consideration of the satisfaction of present desires, the opportunities for future satisfaction, and the possibility of developing or regaining the capacity for self-determination. [President's Commission for the Study of Ethical Problems in Medicine. *Deciding to Forego Life-Sustaining Treatment: A Report on the Ethical, Medical and Legal Issues in Treatment Decisions.* Washington, D.C.: Government Printing Office, 1983, p. 135.]

### 3.0.4 Objective Criteria for Quality of Life

Quality-of-life evaluations, whether personal or observer, are subjective in the sense that they reflect the personal beliefs and values, the likes and dislikes, of the one making the judgment. The question is whether there are any objective criteria against which value judgments can be measured and/or about which all persons would agree. This is a philosophical question of great complexity. For the purposes of clinical judgment we assume that no definitive answer is available. But we suggest that broad, if not universal, agreement would be possible on the following descriptions:

(a) *Restricted quality of life* is an appropriate objective description of a situation in which a person suffers from severe deficits of physical or mental health, that is, the person's functional abilities depart from the normal range found in humans. This is a judgment that might be made by the one who lives the life or by others who observe that person. Clearly, as noted above, the evaluation by the observer and by the one living the life may differ. So, Mr. Cope, the diabetic, who has multiple medical problems, considers his life worthwhile, while observers may judge otherwise.

(b) *Minimal quality of life* is an appropriate objective description for the situation in which a patient or an observer (such as the physician or family member) views one whose general physical condition has greatly deteriorated, whose ability to communicate with others is severely restricted and who suffers discomfort and pain.

*EXAMPLE:* A profoundly demented 85-year-old man, confined to bed with severe arthritis, persistent decubitus ulcers, and diminished respiratory capacity. He must be tube-fed, restrained, and requires opiate analgesia for pain.

(c) *Quality of life below minimal* is an appropriate objective description of the situation in which the patient suffers extreme physical debilitation as well as complete and irreversible loss of sensory and intellectual activity. It might even be suggested that this state would be better described as having no quality, since the ability for personal evaluation has presumably been lost by the person in such a condition. This description applies to persons in a persistent vegetative state (3.2).

*COMMENT:* It is our assumption that few persons would consider either of these latter conditions (b,c) to be good and that those in such conditions would not choose to be in them, if they were able to choose. Many persons, on contemplating these futures for themselves, might say, "I would rather be dead." This is a cautious assumption, since persons seem to judge differently when imagining a situation than they do when actually in such a situation. Still, we address here only the most extreme case, in which a person has permanently lost the ability to interact with the world and with persons. Further, we do not take this assumption alone as the basis for any decision that would lead to the death of the patient: the conditions explained in Chapters 1, 2, and 4 must also be weighed in making a decision about proportionate care (3.4).

## 3.0.5    Divergent Evaluations of Quality of Life

Since evaluation of quality of life is so subjective, different observers will rate certain forms of living quite differently. This can introduce bias and even discrimination into judgments and may affect clinical care adversely. Four major problems of this sort appear in clinical ethics: (a) lack of understanding about the patient's own values; (b) divergence between physicians' assessment of patients' quality of life and the assessments made by patients themselves; (c) bias and discrimination that negatively affect the physician's dedication to the patient's welfare; (d) the introduction of social worth criteria into quality-of-life judgments.

Studies have shown that physicians consistently rate the quality of life of their patients lower than the patients themselves do.

In one study, physicians and patients were asked independently to evaluate living with certain chronic conditions, such as arthritis, ischemic heart disease, chronic pulmonary disease, and cancer. Physicians judged life with these conditions to be less tolerable than did the patients who suffered from them. Physicians based their assessments primarily on disease conditions whereas patients also took into account nonmedical factors such as interpersonal relationships, finances, and social conditions. Also, studies have shown that physicians' quality-of-life assessments do influence important clinical decisions such as those about resuscitation. [Pearlman R, Uhlmann R. Quality of life in chronic disease: perceptions of elderly patients. *J Gerontol* 1988; 43:1125; Starr T, Pearlman R, Uhlmann R. Quality of life and resuscitation decisions in elderly patients. *J Gen Intern Med* 1986; 1:373.]

*EXAMPLE:*   A 62-year-old man with metastatic colon cancer has been doing relatively well until he presents with uremia secondary to obstructive nephropathy. He is encephalopathic. The physician believes that uremia is a quiet way to die, while advancing metastatic disease would be very distressing. He recommends that the obstruction not be relieved. The patient's wife insists on surgical treatment. The patient recovered and lived an additional ten months with satisfactory quality of life until two weeks before his death.

*COMMENT:*   This sort of divergence in evaluation can lead to serious misjudgments about the appropriateness of therapy. It is essential that physicians raise the issue of quality of life with the patient and seek to render as explicit as possible the values held by the patient. Physicians should become more adept in discussing these elusive matters with patients: use of "values histories" may be useful. [Gibson JM. National Values History Project. *Generations* 1990; Supplement, 51–64.]

## 3.0.6   The Repugnant Patient

In 2.9, several patients were described who had characteristics that made it difficult to care for them. Mr. Cope was uncooperative, alcoholic, and unpleasant. Another patient was an abusive drug addict. A third was a habitual criminal. Physicians may find such patients exasperating and even repugnant. This reaction may distort clinical decisions about such patients and affect the quality of life care provided to them. Providers should make strenuous efforts to overcome their negative attitudes toward such patients.

*EXAMPLE:* Mr. C.D. is an alcoholic who inhabits building excavations. He is extremely filthy, foul-mouthed, and, at times, violent and disruptive. He appears quite regularly at the hospital in need of various sorts of care for pneumonia, frostbite, delirium tremens, and so forth. One of the house officers, despite a reprimand from the chief resident, persists in calling him Gomer the Gopher. He is brought to the ER for the third time in a month with bleeding esophageal varices. The ER intern says, "High quality of life like Gomer's we can do without."

*COMMENT:* Mr. C.D.'s quality of life, while certainly low in terms of the values of our culture, is not relevant to medical decisions. He does, however, impose certain burdens on his providers and on society. This contextual factor is considered in Chapter 4.

### 3.0.7  Developmental Disability

Quality-of-life judgments are sometimes made about persons whose lives are limited as a result of developmental disability. Given the range of possibilities for social intercourse, intellectual achievement, personal accomplishment, and productivity open to most human beings, the lives of these persons seem severely restricted. It might be said, then, that they live lives of restricted or minimal quality, in the sense of definitions *a* and *b* in 3.0.4. When decisions about medical care are made for such persons, is such quality of life a relevant consideration?

*EXAMPLE:* Mr. A.T. is a 67-year-old man who has been institutionalized for severe developmental disability since the age of 1 year. His mental age is estimated at less than the 3-year-old level, and his IQ is 10. He develops acute myelogenous leukemia. His guardian says, "His life is of such poor quality. Why should we try to extend it?"

*COMMENT:* The above case recalls one in which an important legal decision was rendered (Saikewicz, 3.3.1). In that case, the court approved a decision not to treat Joseph Saikewicz, a 67-year-old developmentally disabled man, with chemotherapy. However, the court attempted to distinguish between the quality of life of the developmentally disabled, which it did not consider relevant to the decision, and the quality of life that Joseph Saikewicz "was likely to experience" under treatment. Speaking of the continued state of pain and disorientation likely to result from chemotherapy, the courts said, "He would experience fear without the understanding from which other patients draw strength." This distinction suggests a point of ethical importance. Deciding to withhold medical treatment from an individual because that individual belongs to a class of persons whose lives are limited in view of social norms for accomplishment and productivity is ethically dangerous. It looks more to the burden these persons place on society than to the burden these persons themselves experience. The peril of seeing persons as class members for the purpose of medical treatment is the "slippery slope," that is, starting a process in which classes of "undesirables" grow increasingly wider and sweep in more and more persons who are "burdens to themselves and others." This argument is discussed at 4.0.7.

### 3.0.8 Bias and Discrimination

One of the important ethical achievements of medicine in the tradition of Western culture is the tenet that those in need should be cared for regardless of race, religion, or nationality. However, individual physicians may have beliefs and values that lead to biased and discriminatory judgments against certain persons or classes of persons. These judgments may affect clinical decisions. Sometimes these attitudes are explicit: the history of American medicine is stained by discrimination against African-Americans and Native Americans. Today these biases may be less explicit but no less harmful. It is ethically important that they be identified and eliminated from clinical decisions.

(a) *Bias Against the Elderly and the Disabled.* Studies have revealed that many physicians, particularly younger ones, are biased against elderly patients. They are reluctant to deal with them and sometimes make prejudicial judgments about them. [Strain J. Ageism in the medical profession. *Geriatrics* 1981; 36:151.]

*CASE:* An elderly woman is brought unconscious to the emergency department. Paramedics report that her nephew said she was 92 years old. On examination, she is unresponsive, dehydrated, hypotensive, and is found to have a urinary tract infection and pulmonary infiltrates possibly due to aspiration. The ER resident believes she has sepsis from a urinary tract source, but wonders whether to start antibiotics and fluid resuscitation, due to her reported age. The attending physician orders treatment. On recovery, the patient returns to her previous rather vigorous and alert quality of life, which had not been known to the treating physicians.

*COMMENT:* Treatment decisions should be based on medical need and presumed patient preference. Discrimination against persons based on their chronological age is morally wrong. Even if contribution to society is considered important, it is not, in itself, the criterion of just and fair distribution of social benefits. Age is not an accurate indicator of contribution to society. Contribution may be made in many ways other than economic productivity, and present social goods are built on past contributions.

(b) *Life-Style Bias.* Studies have revealed that physicians are no more free of bias against certain life-styles than the general population. In particular, negative attitudes or discomfort at homosexual identity has been noted. One 1987 study showed that, in a sample of physicians, a significant number of physicians stigmatized patients identified as gay and showed less willingness to interact even in ordinary conversation with them. This bias can seriously affect the care of homosexual men with HIV infection and AIDS. While a decade of experience may have mitigated this bias, some providers may still harbor these attitudes. [Kelly S. Stigmatization of AIDS patients by physicians. *Am J Pub Health* 1987; 77:789.]

(c) *Gender Bias.* Gender bias exists, overtly or covertly, throughout our society. In health care, it has been demonstrated that male physicians, quite unconsciously, discount women's health complaints and that research has been designed in ways that fail to evaluate appropriately treatments for women.

(d) *Social Worth.* Judgments about quality of life should be directed primarily to the characteristics and experiences of individuals. However, it is easy to include in such judgments beliefs about how persons with a certain quality of life contribute, or fail to contribute, to the social community of which they are a part. This may be legitimate or it may be extremely prejudicial and unfair.

*EXAMPLE:* Mr. C.D., the homeless and deranged man in 3.0.6, may be thought to have a life of poor quality. He appears to contribute nothing to society and to be, in fact, a burden on social institutions.

*EXAMPLE:* In the early days of renal dialysis, a rationing system was established in which a committee of lay persons was asked to evaluate suitable candidates. They soon found that they were going beyond the personal characteristics of candidates to their contribution to society and using extremely dubious criteria to determine this contribution.

*RECOMMENDATION:* In general, social worth criteria are not relevant to diagnosis and treatment of particular patients. Patients should not be afforded or refused treatment on the basis of social worth. It is not the physician's prerogative to make such judgments in the context of providing medical treatment: criminals, addicts, enemies should be treated in terms of their medical need, not their social worth. However, the impact of a patient's socioeconomic situation may be relevant to prognosis and eligibility for special services such as organ transplantation, and require ability and willingness to undergo rigorous follow-up. Similarly, social worth may be relevant in certain triage situations. On these points, see Chapter 4.

## 3.0.9 P Features of Quality-of-Life Judgments for Infants and Children

Two important differences distinguish these judgments from those in adult care. First, the adult often can express preferences about future states of life and health. Second, when an adult is incapable of expressing preferences, the history of that person's preferences and style of life often allows others to estimate how that person would value and adapt to future states. In pediatrics, the life whose quality is being assessed is almost entirely in the future and no expression of preferences is available. [Arras JD. *Quality of Life in Neonatal Ethics: Beyond Denial and Evasion.*

*Ethical Issues at the Outset of Life.* London: Blackwell Scientific Publications, 1987; Imperiled Newborns. Special Issue. *Hastings Center Report* 1987; 17.]

**Case I.**   Peter, a 12-year-old boy with Down's syndrome, has had a congenital heart lesion, known since birth. No surgical intervention was recommended until his 12th year. Peter's IQ tests at the higher end of the range common to Down's syndrome. He is now a Boy Scout, active in sports, and an average performer in special school. His parents refuse permission for surgery that would effect normal longevity, saying that after they died, his quality of life would be intolerable.

**Case II.**   A newborn infant is noted to have the stigmata of Down's syndrome which is confirmed by chromosome studies. He also suffers from duodenal atresia, for which immediate surgery is indicated. His parents refuse permission, saying that the baby was better dead than living the life of a retarded person.

*COMMENT:*   The perils of quality-of-life judgment are demonstrated in these cases. In Case I, the judgment is about a far future and does not reflect Peter's relative success in dealing with his limitation. The judgment of Peter's parents does not reflect significant facts about their son's life and, at the same time, has implications of great consequence and certain outcome for their son. Deprived of the recommended surgery, he will continue to live for some time and slowly develop the debilitating effects of severe cardiac insufficiency and pulmonary hypertension. In Case II, a general predisposition to disvalue limited intelligence, achievement, productivity, and independence colors judgment. These social values, while highly valued in our culture, are not the only human values. They are not so important that their invocation should lead to death for those who can attain them in only limited degree. Questions raised by the social problems of providing appropriate care and education are discussed in Chapter 4.

*RECOMMENDATION:*   Medical interventions that are generally effective in alleviating physical disability are ethically mandatory when the only supposed contraindication is developmental disabilities in the range characteristic of Down's syndrome. More complicated medical conditions, such as major cardiac deformity, may be genuine contraindications, but for the same reasons that they may contraindicate surgery for an otherwise normal infant.

## 3.0.10P Best Interest Standard

Children have no history of preferences on which to base a surrogate judgment. Thus, the first standard for surrogate decisions, substituted judgment, is not relevant; all surrogate judgments for minor children must adhere to the best interest standard (2.7.2, 3.0.3).

**Case I.** Monica, born at term, is noted at birth to have a large thoracolumbar myelomeningocele, which is leaking cerebrospinal fluid. In addition to extreme kyphosis, Monica appears to be microcephalic. Computerized tomography of the head shows cerebral dysgenesis and ventriculomegaly, with a cortical mantle of less than 5 mm. Monica's parents, who understand the situation, request that no medical interventions be performed. They wish to take Monica home to die.

**Case II.** An 1,100-gram premature male infant, born at 32 weeks gestational age, is now 2 days old and in the recovery phase of moderately severe hyaline membrane disease. A drop in hematocrit and a prolonged indirect hyperbilirubinemia suggest occult bleeding. A cranial ultrasound study confirms a grade III intraventricular hemorrhage. After being informed of the possible risks of mental retardation, the infant's parents request that the mechanical ventilation be stopped.

**Case III.** John is a 2-day-old infant who was started on a prostaglandin infusion when an echocardiogram confirmed that a hypoplastic left heart was the cause of his poor pulses. In order to control respiratory distress, John was intubated, ventilated and sedated. The neonatologists are pleased with how John has stabilized in response to their management. They discuss the various options with John's parents. This intelligent young couple begin by saying they want John to have as normal a life as possible, but express their concern about putting him through suffering to achieve it.

*COMMENT:*   In Case I, the prognosis includes severe deformity of the spine and lower limbs, incontinence of bowel and bladder, and the near certainty of profound mental retardation. Multiple surgical procedures will be required during early life for orthopedic problems, and there is high likelihood of frequent infection of bladder catheter and ventriculoperitoneal shunt. Monica will never be able to understand and communicate. The combination of extreme and painful disabilities and severe retardation constitutes a quality of life that can confidently be judged to be undesirable for, and undesired by, any human being.

In Case II, there is significant probability of disability, although the extent is unpredictable. There may be some residual chronic lung deficiencies. The difference lies in the predictability, as in Case I, of a life of physical pain without even the solace of experiencing the compassion of others and of understanding one's own condition, as contrasted with an uncertain prediction of mental or physical limitation only in Case II. The judgment of quality of life in the first invokes a condition that can confidently be evaluated as one that any human being would wish to avoid. The situation described in Case II affords no such confidence. The criteria for judging treatment to be in the child's best interest are more applicable to Case II than to Case I.

In Case III, there are only three options for John's care. Since a hypoplastic left heart is incompatible with life, the parents may choose to allow John to die. They may, however, choose a staged surgical repair of the heart, known as the Norwood procedure. Currently, some two-thirds of infants survive up to five years after three operations performed over the first three years of life. At the same time, many of these infants suffer from major developmental disabilities as complications of surgery or hospitalization. A final option is heart transplantation, but the long wait, due to the shortage of organs, makes this an unlikely option.

*RECOMMENDATION:*   We propose that a decision to refrain from intervention that is designed to prolong life is ethically justified in Case I, but not in Case II. The federal Baby Doe Rules state that life-sustaining treatment is not mandatory when "the provision of such treatment would be virtually futile in terms of the survival of the infant and the treatment itself under such circumstances would be inhumane" (At 14888). In Case III, the parents have the discretion to choose or not to choose the surgery. We suggest that parents make a reasonable choice in not choosing the Norwood procedure. At the same time, their choice of the procedure would be defensible. The suffering and disabilities imposed by the treatment itself on an infant, with limited prospects for survival and a healthy life even with the procedure, justify their decision to refrain. Parental desire to save their child from certain death gives support to their choice. The obligation to alleviate pain, suffering and disability is as serious as an obligation to save an endangered life. No moral obligation is imposed on anyone to assist in the perpetuation of such a life in the absence of a request from the one who lives it. [American Academy of Pediatrics, Guidelines on Foregoing Life-sustaining Medical Treatment. *Pediatrics* 1994; 93:532–536; Campbell AGM, Kuhse H, Quality of life, and Stahlman M, Weir R. Withholding and withdrawing therapy. In: Goldworth A. et al., eds. *Ethics and Perinatology*. New York: Oxford University Press, 1995.]

## 3.1                    ENHANCING QUALITY OF LIFE

Medical interventions are aimed at improving quality of life for patients. Even interventions with this beneficial purpose sometimes raise ethical problems.

### 3.1.1  Rehabilitation

Rehabilitation medicine aims at an improvement in quality of life, demonstrated by restoration of mobility, ability to work, and independent living. The autonomy of the patient is a primary goal, and the preferences and values of the patient define the goal; the cooperation of the patient is crucial. In this setting, several special ethical problems predominate. These problems sometimes arise because the patient's preferences and judgment of personal quality of life conflict with the physiatrist's medical knowledge and values.

*EXAMPLE:*   A program of rehabilitation is recommended to the gymnastics instructor described in 3.0.3. He initially refuses to participate in such a program, stating, "I'm crippled and the quality of my life is so bad that it can't be improved." The rehabilitation team has a quite different view of his possibilities. They invite him to continue to discuss the issues and propose some short-term goals.

*COMMENT:* This case could be discussed in Chapter 2, since it is an instance of problems arising around patient preferences. However, quality of life is central to the physiatrist's evaluation of whether the patient's wishes should be honored. Rehabilitation medicine stresses an educational framework for treatment: persons are taught skills and taught to live within the limits of inevitable disabilities. Similarly, ethical problems regarding appropriate treatment should be first addressed as educational issues: the physician attempts to aid the patient to understand the problem in as full a context as possible. [EB: "Rehabilitation Medicine," IV, 2201-2206; Ethical and Policy Issues in Rehabilitation Medicine. Special Issue. *Hastings Center Report* 1987; 17; Scofield GR. Ethical considerations in rehabilitation medicine. *Arch Phys Med Rehabil* 1993; 74:341.]

### 3.1.2 Pain Relief and Palliative Care

The quality of life of terminally ill patients is enhanced by palliative care which includes skilled application of pain-relieving drugs. Unfortunately, skilled use of pain-relieving drugs remains a rare talent in medical practice. This failure, however, is increasingly recognized, and several new approaches are promising. They include research on pain and suffering, improved teaching and training for physicians and residents, and the emergence of several specialty fields, including pain medicine and palliative care medicine. The hospice approach provides many techniques for palliative care and should always be considered for terminally ill patients.

Patients should not be kept on a regimen inadequate to control pain because of the ignorance of the physician or because of an ungrounded fear of addiction. Medical licensing boards in all states are extremely cautious about physicians' abuse of their authority to prescribe drugs and sometimes carry that caution to the point where their oversight inhibits appropriate medication for pain. Local medical societies, in collaboration with academic medical centers, should attempt to assist the licensing boards toward a balanced policy in this matter.

Attempts to achieve adequate relief of pain have another side effect, namely, the clouding of the patient's consciousness and the hindering of the patient's communication with family and friends. This double effect may be ethically troubling to physicians and nurses. In such situations no ethical principle will resolve the problem. Rather, sensitive attention to the patient's needs, together with skilled medical management, should lead as close as possible to the desired objective: maximum relief of pain with minimal diminution of consciousness and communication. Of course, if the patient is able to express preferences, these should be followed.

Efforts to relieve pain by opiates entail the risk of respiratory depression, leading to death. It is clear that relief of pain is one of the major goals of medicine, and it often is heartily desired by the patient. On occasion, it is difficult to manage pain medication so that pain palliation and respiratory depression are balanced. In such situations, should maintenance of adequate respiratory status take precedence over pain relief? Relief of pain and maintenance of function are both goals of medicine. However, when the goal of prolonging life can no longer be attained, the relief of pain becomes the primary goal to be sought during the remaining time of the patient's life. Pain medications, like most drugs, entail risks, and in the face of imminent death, a dosage regimen with higher risks than would otherwise be tolerated is rational. [EB: "Hospice and End of Life Care," II, 1157–1160.]

### 3.1.3 Double Effect

The ethics of this problem are sometimes discussed in terms of the principle of "double effect." While this ethical thesis has been much criticized, many ethicists find the following arguments acceptable.

On occasion, persons are faced with a decision that cannot be avoided and that, in the circumstances, will cause both desirable and undesirable effects. These effects are inextricably linked. One of those effects is intended by the agent and is ethically permissible (e.g., relief of pain is a benefit); the other is not intended by the agent and is ethically undesirable (e.g., risk of respiratory depression is a harm). Proponents of this argument state that an ethically permissible effect can be allowed, even if the ethically undesirable one will inevitably follow, when the following conditions are present:

(a) The action itself is ethically good or at least indifferent, that is, neither good nor evil in itself (in this case the action is the administration of a drug, a morally indifferent act).

(b) The agent must intend the good effects, not the evil effects, even though these are foreseen (in this case the intention is to relieve pain, not to compromise respiration).

(c) The morally objectionable effect cannot be a means to the morally permissible one (in this case respiratory compromise is not the means to relief of pain).

In this argument the major practical problem for the clinician lies with the second condition (b), since often the intention of the physician is mixed: to relieve pain and to hasten death. If it can be said that the dosages administered are clinically rational, that is, no more drug is administered than is necessary for adequate pain relief, the intention to relieve pain seems primary and the action is ethical. If doses in excess of clinical necessity are given, the intention to hasten death seems primary. Respiratory depression is the probable side effect of appropriate dosages of morphine (i.e., sufficient to relieve pain). It is "unintended" in the sense that, if pain could be relieved by other means which would not have the effect, those means would be preferred. If this latter intention becomes primary, the action would be judged unethical. Roman Catholic medical ethics employs this argument to justify clinically appropriate pain medication for relief of pain, even if the unintended foreseen effect is the shortening of the patient's life. [EB: "Double Effect," II, 636–641; PBE: "Intended Effects vs. Merely Foreseen Effects," 206–211; Double effect: theoretical function and bioethical implications. *J Med Philos* 1991; 16(5).]

**Case I.** Mrs. Comfort suffers from carcinoma of the breast with lymphangitic spread to lungs and bony metastases. She requires increasing narcotic dosage for relief of pain. Her pulmonary function deteriorates so that her $P_{O_2}$ is 45 and $P_{CO_2}$ is 55 when she is pain-free. Mrs. Comfort is now receiving two tablets of 15 mg slow-release morphine every 4 hours. She asks for further morphine. Her physician hesitates, fearing that further medication, given her already compromised respiratory ability, will cause Mrs. Comfort's death. However, he orders 30 mg of oral morphine every 2 h.

**Case II.** A 63-year-old terminally ill woman, with widely metastatic esophageal cancer and profound malnutrition, develops peritonitis from a leaking gastrostomy tube. Attempted surgical correction of the leak was unsuccessful and she continued to have peritonitis with severe abdominal pain. The patient and her family decide to have a morphine drip for control of pain. The dose of morphine is titrated to the patient's pain and to maintain her ability to communicate with her family. She experiences some decrease in respiratory drive and mental alertness. Six days after the morphine drip was started, the patient is no longer responsive. Her husband asks whether the inevitable could not be hastened. The attending physician himself dials up the morphine to 20 mg/h. The patient lapses into coma. She dies 12 hours later.

*COMMENT:* These two cases illustrate the application of the principle of double effect. The morphine drip is administered in response to pain with the knowledge that it increases the risk of respiratory depression. In Case I, the dosage is maintained at a level needed to achieve a pain-free state. In Case II, the dosage, at first rational, was increased to a point at which death was clearly intended. In that case, the ethical problem of euthanasia is raised. This is discussed in 3.5.

### 3.1.4 Psychological, Social, and Spiritual Relief of Suffering

Relief of pain is a medical goal sought by medication, surgery, and rehabilitation, but pain is often only one component of a psychological, social, and spiritual phenomenon usually called suffering. Concentration on the physiological components of pain through pharmacological or surgical interventions, without equal attention to the psychological, social, and spiritual, may bring little relief. Even if relief is achieved in the physiological sense, other important ethical responsibilities may be left unfulfilled, for example, aiding patients to deal with their death and its effect on others. Physicians should make themselves aware of these components and seek assistance from those expert in dealing with them. The presence of religious counselors is often of immeasurable value to the patient, to the family, and to the physician.

### 3.2 QUALITY OF LIFE BELOW MINIMAL

Quality-of-life discussions often take place in situations where an ethical decision must be made about continuing life-supporting interventions for a patient who is unable to express any personal preferences or whose expression is indiscernible or indecipherable as the result of mental incapacity. In addition, physicians may suspect that, if some suggested intervention succeeds, the patient will survive, but with severe deficits of physical or mental capacity. The question is then asked, "Is such a life worth living? In this sense, raising the issue of quality of life seems equivalent to wondering whether no life at all is better than a life with severe deficits. While this is a difficult philosophical question,the pressure of clinical decisions demand a practical resolution: the following sections suggest some consideration appropriate to clinical decisions of this sort. [ME: ch. 12, 363–394; Weir R. *Abating Treatment with Critically Ill Patients.* New York: Oxford University Press, 1989.]

**Case.**    Mrs. Care, the patient with multiple sclerosis, is living at home. She has a respiratory arrest associated with gram-negative pneumonia and septicemia. She is rushed to the hospital and placed on a respirator. After two weeks, Mrs. Care has not recovered consciousness; a neurology consultant states that Mrs. Care has the neurological signs consistent with persistent vegetative state. At no time in the course of her care has she expressed any clear preferences about her future. Should respiratory support be continued?

*COMMENT:*    (a) Mrs. Care is not brain dead in the proper sense of having lost all function of both higher and lower brain. She still has brainstem activity, respiration, and heartbeat. Thus, she is not legally dead (1.5).

(b) Persistent vegetative state is a neurological diagnosis defined as "a sustained, complete loss of self-aware cognition with wake/sleep cycles and other autonomic functions remaining relatively intact. The condition can either follow acute, severe bilateral cerebral damage or develop gradually as the end stage of a progressive dementia." Studies show that, when properly diagnosed, recovery of consciousness is almost unprecedented. The majority of these patients will not require respiratory support, but will require artificial nutrition. Since persons in PVS retain some reflex activities, they may have some eye movement, swallowing, grimacing, and pupillary adjustment to light. This is naturally quite disturbing to observers, leading them to hold out much more hope for recovery than is actually warranted by the clinical facts. Medical interventions promise no benefit beyond sustaining organic life. [The Multi-Society Task Force on PVS. Medical aspects of the persistent vegetative state, Part 1. *NEJM* 1994; 330:1499–1508; Part 2. 1994;

330:1572–1579; The Persistent Problem of PVS. *Hastings Center Report* 1988; 18(1):26–47.]

(c) All the functions usual to human interaction and, to the best of the observer's knowledge, all forms of cognitive and sensory experience are absent or extremely deficient. It is highly unlikely that any of these functions will be recovered.

(d) Care must be taken not to mistake persistent vegetative state for another neurological condition known as locked-in state. In this latter condition, lesions in the midbrain paralyze efferent pathways governing movement and communication but leave consciousness intact. Neurological consultation is required to make the differential diagnosis.

(e) Note how this version of the case differs from Mrs. Care's condition as described in 1.2.2–1.2.3, where her death is imminent. In that situation the judgment that further intervention is futile in terms of achieving medical goals justifies the decision to discontinue mechanical support. In this case Mrs. Care is neither dead nor imminently dying. Her MS has not advanced to the point where it can be considered terminal; indeed, at this point, she may have a number of years of life ahead. If her pneumonia resolves and she can be weaned from the respirator, she will not recover from her underlying disease, nor will she return to mental functioning sufficient for communication. Her life, supported by mechanical means, will consist of vegetative activities alone (as far as can be known). On the other hand, if respirator support is removed, Mrs. Care may breathe on her own and continue to live in a persistent vegetative state. Life in a vegetative state seems to the physician and the family a life of lower than minimum—indeed, of no quality. Their hope is that, once the respirator is discontinued, Mrs. Care will die quickly.

*RECOMMENDATION:* In our judgment it is ethically permissible to discontinue respiratory support and all other forms of life-sustaining treatment. We argue that the conjunction of four features of this case justifies such a decision.

(a) In the state of irreversible loss of cognitive and communicative function, the individual no longer has any "interests," that is, nothing that happens to the patient can in any way advance his or her welfare nor can the individual evaluate any event or state that occurs. Thus, if no interests can be served, no interventions are mandatory.

(b) No goals of medicine other than support of organic life are being or will be accomplished. We do not believe that this goal, in and of itself, is an overriding and independent goal of medicine.

(c) None of the other goals of medicine can be attained and thus no other medical benefits accrue to the patient.

(d) No preferences of the patient are known that might contradict the assumption that she would wish organic life continued. The conjunction of these factors justifies the conclusion that physicians have no ethical obligation to continue life-sustaining interventions. Where no interests are served and no goals of medicine are obtainable, no duty exists.

Our conclusion is supported by the Opinion of the Council on Ethical and Judicial Affairs of the AMA (1989): "Even if death is not imminent but a patient is beyond doubt permanently unconscious, and there are adequate safeguards to confirm the accuracy of the diagnosis, it is not unethical to discontinue all means of life-prolonging medical treatment." The President's Commission on the Study of Ethical Problems in Medicine came to the same conclusion. [Council of Scientific Affairs and Council on Ethical and Judicial Affairs of the American Medical Association. Persistent vegetative state and the decision to withdraw or withhold life support. *JAMA* 1990; 263:426; President's Commission, *Deciding to Forego Life-Sustaining Treatment*. Ch. 5. Patients with permanent loss of consciousness. Washington, D.C.: U.S. Government Printing Office, 1983.]

**Case I (Continued).**   Mrs. Care is in a persistent vegetative state. She is not on a respirator. She now becomes anuric and is in renal failure. Should dialysis be initiated?

*COMMENT:*   This version of the case involves an instance of not starting an intervention rather than stopping one already being used. Many interventions are initiated at times when their use is quite rational. The achievement of important goals is still seen as possible. When these goals cannot be achieved, and when there are other important considerations, for example, absence of patient preference and quality of life below the minimal, they may be discontinued. Some believe that there is an ethical difference between starting and stopping: the former being more permissible than the latter. There may be psychological or emotional differences: Some physicians find it more troubling to stop an ongoing intervention than not to initiate a new one. The initiation of treatment expresses some measure of hope and assuages the uncertainty that besets clinical medicine. If, despite the physician's efforts, the patient succumbs to the disease, the physician has tried and done her best. However, in withdrawing or stopping treatment, the physician may feel responsible (in a causal sense) for the events that follow, even though she bears no responsibility (in the sense of ethical or legal accountability) either for the disease process or for the patient's succumbing to the disease.

Finally, after deciding to refrain from aggressive therapeutic efforts, new medical problems, such as infection or renal failure, sometimes tempt physicians to initiate therapeutic interventions to deal with these particular problems. This is, of course, irrational, unless the intervention has as its purpose another goal more appropriate to the situation, such as providing comfort to the dying patient.

*RECOMMENDATION:* The decision to forgo support is justified in both versions of Mrs. Care's case. It is the common position of medical ethicists, supported by many judicial decisions, that the distinction between stopping and starting is neither ethically nor legally relevant. It is our position that there is no significant ethical difference between stopping and starting if the essential considerations regarding medical indications, patient preference, and quality of life are the same.

### 3.2.1   Orders Not to Resuscitate and Quality of Life

The DNAR order, discussed in 1.3 in terms of futility, is sometimes contemplated in conditions of quality of life below minimal. A DNAR order may be written when the patient, advised that a successful resuscitation would provide at best a seriously impaired quality of life, requests or accepts a recommendation for nonresuscitation. In such cases, the expressed preferences of the patient are essential. If the patient is incapable of expressing a preference, a physician may recommend a DNAR order to the surrogate on the same grounds. The surrogate should consider the recommendation in accord with the standards for surrogate judgment (2.7). Finally, in emergent situations, when no surrogate is available, a physician may write a DNAR order based on prognosis of seriously impaired quality of life only when convinced that, even if resuscitated, the patient is likely to die soon thereafter or on the basis of sound evidence that resulting life would be below minimal quality.

## 3.2.2   Minimal Quality of Life

In the above cases, Mrs. Care's condition, a persistent vegetative state, represents a quality of life falling below what we have called "lower than minimal." In such situations, the ethical justification for refraining from medical intervention seems to us quite strong. However, in other cases, quality of life, although an important consideration, is much less definitive as the ethical justification of a decision to refrain from intervention.

**Case I.**   Mr. B.R. is 84 years old and living in a nursing home. He was diagnosed as having Alzheimer's dementia five years ago. He is chairbound, does not respond meaningfully to human attention, but is often very agitated. He cannot now express, nor had he previously expressed, preferences regarding care. He is otherwise physically healthy. He is difficult to feed, frequently choking and expelling food. He has been treated several times in the past month for aspiration pneumonia with antibiotics and fluids. During the night he develops a violent cough and wheezing. He has a fever of 100. The visiting physician diagnoses aspiration pneumonia. Should he be treated again?

**Case II.**   Mrs. A.W., a 34-year-old woman, married with three children, has had a long history of scleroderma and ischemic ulcerations of fingers and toes. She is admitted with early renal failure. The big toe of her right foot and several fingers of her left hand became gangrenous. Several days later she consents to amputation of the right foot and the thumb and first finger of her left hand. After surgery she is alternately obtunded and confused. She develops pneumonia and is placed on a respirator. The remaining fingers of her left hand become gangrenous and more extensive amputation is required. Her renal condition worsens, and it is now necessary to consider initiating dialysis. The attending says, "How could anyone want to live a life of such terrible quality?" Should the respirator be discontinued? Should dialysis be initiated?

*COMMENT:*   In Mr. B.R.'s case, quality of life refers to the observer's assessment in view of low levels of physical and mental activity. Nothing is known about Mr. B.R.'s own subjective experience. Mr. B.R. will suffer recurring episodes of aspiration. Use of feeding tubes will probably entail restraints due to Mr. B.R.'s frequent agitation. Quality of life, then, has become a relevant consideration, but only insofar as it refers to an objective state, particularly inability to control motor activities and to cooperate with care in any way. Mr. B.R.'s chronological age is not, in itself, a reason to refrain from treating; only insofar as his chronological age correlates with this physiological state does it become relevant. This objective state makes achievement of medical goals increasingly impossible at the same time medical problems continue to arise. In this case, considerations of futility as well as quality of life are relevant. On the other hand, the severe physical deficits and problems of rehabilitation faced by Mrs. A.W. evoke in the observer an assessment that "no one would want to live that way." This, of course, cannot be verified by Mrs. A.W. at this time. Mrs. A.W. has multiple problems, but all are potentially reversible, with the exception of the loss of extremities. In addition, she herself has consented to the initial amputations, suggesting her willingness to live with these deficits. Finally, her vital personality prior to her surgery suggested to the staff that she had the ability to cope with rehabilitation and the difficulties of subsequent life.

*RECOMMENDATION:*   In our opinion it is ethically permissible to refrain from treating Mr. B.R.'s pneumonia after several episodes have shown this to be the beginning of a recurring pattern. Thus, it is ethically permissible to refrain from treatment of pneumonia, permitting this disease to be, as it was once called, "the old man's friend." There is no obligation to proceed with measures such as gastronomy or gastrogavage, which would require the insult of permanent constraint and increase the risk of infection. On the other hand, it is ethically obligatory to continue to treat Mrs. A.W.: significant medical goals can still be attained, and although her current preferences cannot be ascertained, it can be presumed that she favors continued treatment.

### 3.2.3   Nutrition and Hydration

Mrs. Care has been started on intravenous fluids and nutrients. Is it permissible to discontinue these measures after she is

judged to be in persistent vegetative state? Mr. B.R. has deteriorated mentally and now lies in fetal position, showing no
response to verbal or tactile stimuli. Should a feeding tube be
employed? In both cases, death would ensue from starvation
and dehydration unless artificial means are used. Is there any
special obligation to employ these measures that distinguishes
them from respiratory support or mediation? [PBE: "Sustenance
Technologies vs. Medical Technologies," 202–206; Lynn J. *By No
Extraordinary Means: The Choice to Forego Life-Sustaining Food
and Water.* Bloomington, Ind: University of Indiana Press, 1986;
Dresser RS, Boisaubin E. Ethics, law and nutritional support.
*Arch Intern Med* 1985; 145:122.]

*COMMENT:*    There has been considerable disagreement on
this issue. Some authors argue that feeding is so basic a human
function and so symbolic of care that it constitutes "ordinary
means" and should never be forgone. They also note that forgoing these techniques is a direct cause of death. They wonder
about the social implications of a policy that would deprive the
most helpless of basic human attention. Other ethicists judge
that the burdens of continual life of pain, discomfort, immobil-
ity, dimmed consciousness, and loss of communication would
not be desired by any human, and those burdens so overwhelm
benefits of life that there is no obligation to assist in sustaining
life. This measure, like all other medical interventions, should
be judged in view of the proportion of burdens over benefits.
The circumstances that justify the decision to forgo feeding are:
no significant medical goal other than maintenance of organic
life is possible, the patient is so mentally incapacitated that no
preferences can be expressed now or in the future, no prior
preferences for continued sustenance in such a situation have
been expressed, and the patient's situation is such that no discomfort or pain will be experienced. Given the diversity of
opinion, we judge that either position is ethically permissible,
but prefer the opinion that, like all other medical interventions,
the ethical propriety of nutrition and hydration should be evaluated in light of the principle of proportionality (3.4).

*RECOMMENDATION:*    It is ethically permissible to forgo
nutrients and hydration in Mrs. Care's case. She is in a persistent
vegetative state and, presumably, lacks all experience. She will
not experience discomfort from starvation or dehydration. In Mr.

B.R.'s case, opinion would be more divided. Some commentators might note that, while profoundly demented, he is still capable of experience: indeed, his continual moaning and restlessness indicate that he is uncomfortable. If, then, discontinuing nutrients and fluids would aggravate his distress, it should not be done. It is unlikely that severe pain or discomfort follows the withdrawal of nutrient support in a patient so deteriorated and likely that death will occur rather quickly. Thus, it is our opinion, that nutrition and hydration may be discontinued. Mr. B.R. should be kept as comfortable as possible.

**3.3**                          **LEGAL IMPLICATIONS**

The death of a patient resulting from a decision to discontinue medical intervention on the grounds of quality of life has legal implications. In the cases described in these sections, the patient could be kept alive, perhaps for some time, by continued use of the respirator, by dialysis, or in some other way. It is the "quality" of that continued life that leads to the decision to cease intervention. In contrast, the cases of termination of treatment discussed tin Chapter 1 involved persons whose death was imminent and for whom further intervention was unlikely to attain medical goals. The cases in Chapter 2 dealt with termination of treatment which a competent patient had declined. Cases of both sorts are not likely to generate legal problems unless someone, such as a relative or another physician, claims the judgment of medical futility was wrongly made or that the patient's preferences were ignored. Cases where quality of life is the central issue are more legally problematic: A person who could be kept alive is allowed to die. In legal theory this might be considered homicide (although the traditional definitions of homicide certainly did not envision the problems occasioned by modern medical technology). The physician might be accused of murder, criminal negligence, or named as an accomplice in the illegal decision of another if he or she accedes to or does not object to the discontinuing of life-support by another. To our knowledge, physicians have been criminally charged with homicide for discontinuing nutrition and hydration in only one such case. (*Barber v. Superior Court*, 3.3.1). Charges in this case were dismissed by an appellate court before any trial was held. Nevertheless, fear of such possibilities, coupled with conservative legal advice, often causes physicians to hesitate in making decisions of this sort. However, in many important legal cases, courts have given approval to decisions to withhold or terminate life-support. In the Karen Ann Quinlan case (3.3.1), first of these cases to be adjudicated, the court wrote, "no compelling interest of the State could compel Karen to endure the unendurable, only to vegetate a few measurable months with no realistic possibility of returning to any semblance of cognitive or sapient life." The only case of this sort to reach the United States Supreme Court (Cruzan, 3.3.1), did not deny the relevance of quality of life argument, but supported the legal provision in the state of Missouri that requires "clear and convincing evidence" of the patient's preferences. This ruling allows other states to establish different standards. Many courts, including the U. S. Supreme Court, do not exclude artificial nutrition and hydration from the life-sustaining treatments that can be omitted. The legal arguments in these cases are complex and controversial. Although the courts have been reluctant to base decisions on "quality-of-life" grounds, the legal perplexities are being resolved to some extent.

*RECOMMENDATION:* In cases of this sort, it is our opinion that physicians are acting within the law, as currently understood, when they recommend that life-supporting interventions be withheld or withdrawn, unless there is specific law to the contrary in any particular jurisdiction. The conditions required for this decision are: (a) it is virtually certain that further medical intervention will not attain any of the goals of medicine other than sustaining organic life, (b) the preferences of the patient are not known and cannot be expressed, (c) quality of life clearly falls below minimal, (d) family are in accord. We hold this opinion because, despite the legal perplexities, most leading cases thus far adjudicated have affirmed the legal correctness of allowing the patient to die when these conditions are present. In addition, we consider it advisable for institutions to establish an appropriate review committee for cases that present problems (4.10). Finally, institutions should request their legal counsels to prepare clear instructions for the medical staff in view of prevailing local law.

### 3.3.1  Judicial Decisions

The most important judicial decisions relevant to cases of this sort are summarized below. These summaries are brief and, given the legal complexities, are provided only to familiarize the reader with the names of the cases and the principal issues.

Fuller description and the proper legal citations can be found in many places. [See, for example, Meisel A. *The Right to Die*. New York: Wiley and Sons, 1989; Supplement 1992; Meyers DW. *Medico-Legal Implications of Death and Dying*. San Francisco: Bancroft-Whitney, 1981; Supplement 1991; *Current Opinions with Annotations of the Ethical and Judicial Council of the American Medical Association*. Chicago: AMA, Issued annually.]

**Judicial Decisions Relating to Life-Supporting Interventions.** *In the Matter of Shirley Dinnerstein* (Mass. App. Ct., 1978.) Upheld validity of "no-code" order on 67-year-old woman suffering from Alzheimer's disease and ruled that such orders did not need court approval.

*Application of Eichner* (Fox) (New York App. Ct., 1980). Trial court authorized guardian of 83-year-old religious brother in "irreversible vegetative state" to request that respirator be discontinued, based on evidence of patient's wishes. Appellate court affirmed and laid out procedures to be followed in future cases.

*In re Quinlan* (N.J. Sup. Jud. Ct., 1976). Authorized discontinuance of respirator for 21-year-old comatose woman in permanent vegetative state, based on her constitutional right of privacy as asserted by her parents on her behalf. Stated patient would not return to "conscious and sapient condition."

*Superintendent of Belchertown State School v. Saikewicz* (Mass. Sup. Ct., 1977). Affirmed trial court decision not to order chemotherapy on a 67-year-old severely retarded and institutionalized man suffering from acute myeloblastic leukemia, also on right to privacy grounds, but stressed the role of courts in reviewing such questions.

*In the Matter of Spring* (Mass. Sup. Jud. Ct., 1980). Upheld right of 77-year-old man who was senile and suffered from kidney disease to stop hemodialysis. The Supreme Court emphasized that this was not a decision to be delegated to the attending physician, and the man's wife and son, but rather must be made by the probate court on appropriate findings.

*Barber v. Superior Court* (Cal. App. Ct., 1983). The court ruled that not only may a respirator be removed from an irreversibly comatose patient but also it is permissible in certain circumstances to discontinue fluids and nutrition. A medical determination that it would be appropriate to withdraw such life-support must be made in each case. The incompetent patient's guardian or next-of-kin may then authorize the withdrawal. In this case, the two attending physicians were indicted on homicide charges, but the appeals court dismissed the charges before trial.

*Bartling v. Superior Court* (Cal. App. Ct., 1984). Affirmed right of a 70-year-old man suffering from multiple chronic, serious illnesses to refuse all medical treatment, even life-sustaining, based on California constitutional right of privacy. The patient was competent and explicitly requesting discontinuance of ventilator support against hospital refusal. The right to have life support equipment disconnected is not limited to comatose, terminally ill patients, or representatives acting on their behalf.

*In re Conroy* (New Jersey Sup. Ct., 1985). The legal guardian for an 84-year-old severely demented woman sought to have all life-sustaining medical treatment, including feeding tubes, withdrawn. The court ruled that life-sustaining treatment may be withdrawn if it would be in the incompetent patient's best interest, that is, the pain and suffering of continued existence outweigh the benefits derived from prolonged life.

*In re Jobes* (New Jersey Sup. Ct., 1987). Upheld right of guardian (husband) of a 31-year-old woman in PVS for five years after vehicular accident to remove feeding tube, based not on evidence of prior wishes, but on irreversible condition.

*Brophy v. New England Sinai Hospital* (Mass. Sup. Jud. Ct., 1986). Wife of 46-year-old man who had suffered ruptured brain aneurysm and was in PVS requested authority to terminate artificial feeding. Court granted authority, noting that state interest in preserving life "encompasses a broader interest than mere corporeal existence."

*In the matter of O'Connor* (New York App. Ct., 1988). Court denied the petition of guardians of a 77-year-old woman to withhold artificial feeding on grounds that patient's prior wishes had not been sufficiently specific.

*In the matter of Cruzan* (U. S. Sup. Ct., 1990). In only termination of treatment case to be reviewed by the U. S. Supreme Court, the right of the state of Missouri to require "clear and convincing evidence" of the patient's prior wishes was upheld. If such evidence was present, artificial feeding was considered medical treatment that could be withheld.

## 3.4                          PROPORTIONATE CARE

The traditional discussions of the ethics of forgoing life-sustaining treatment have turned on certain distinctions, such as omission/commission, withholding/withdrawing, active/passive, and ordinary/

extraordinary care. One still hears in clinical settings such remarks as "withholding treatment might be acceptable, but once it's started, we cannot withdraw," or "would extubation be active or passive?" Recent study has shown these distinctions to be confused and confusing. They are little more than summary statements of elaborate and sometimes faulty arguments, rather than justifications. Unfortunately, these terms are often substitutes for careful attention to details and for analytic thinking. We recommend that decisions to forgo intervention not be based on invocation of these classic distinctions. [PBE: 196–207; ME: Brock DW. "Death and Dying," 363–94; President's Commission, *Deciding to Forego Life-Sustaining Treatment,* Washington, D.C.: Government Printing Office, 1983, The elements of good decision making, ch.3 pp. 43–90.]

In place of these distinctions, the "principle of proportionality" has recently been endorsed by many ethicists. This principle states that a medical treatment is ethically mandatory to the extent that it is likely to confer greater benefits than burdens upon the patient. It is an updated version of one of the distinctions mentioned in the previous paragraph, namely, "ordinary/extraordinary." In recent times, the original meaning of this distinction, which originated in Roman Catholic moral theology, has been obscured. Today it seems to refer to the elaborateness, rarity or investigational nature of a procedure. Originally, it designated the relation or proportion between the expected benefits of treatment and the burdens and disadvantages thereof. Thus, one Catholic theologian wrote:

> Extraordinary means of preserving life are all medicines, treatments, and operations, which cannot be obtained without excessive expense, pain or other inconvenience for the patient or for others, or which, if used, would not offer a reasonable hope of benefit to the patient. [Kelly G. *Medico-Moral Problems.* St. Louis: Catholic Hospital Association, 1958.]

The principle of proportionality, then, expresses this traditional concept: the correct test of the ethical obligation to recommend or provide a medical intervention is the estimate of its promised benefit over its attendant burdens. This test may be applied even when the burden of omitting treatment is the death of patient (which, in fact, may often be seen as a benefit). Although benefit-burden ratios are intrinsic to all medical decision-making, it is important to notice that the principle of proportionality endorses this form of reasoning even in life-death decisions, which had often been thought to exclude such calculation in favor of an absolute duty to preserve life. The principle of proportionality states that no such absolute duty exists: preservation of life is an obligation that binds only when life can be judged more a benefit than a burden by and for the patient.

The principle of proportionality clearly applies to the patient's preferences. Patients have the right to determine what they will accept as benefits and burdens. However, proportionality applies as well to medical indications. Physicians must formulate in their own minds the benefit-burden ratio in order to recommend appropriate options to patients or to their surrogates. The most difficult application of proportionality occurs when surrogates apply this principle to reach decisions for irreversibly incapacitated individuals who have left no prior oral or written directive.

### 3.4.1    Conclusion

Quality of life may be a decisive consideration in a clinical decision to withhold or withdraw interventions necessary for life when the following conditions are present:

(a) The indications of medical treatment are such that the goal of preservation of organic life without attainment of other goals is likely to be the only accomplishment, or the achievement of other medical goals capable of contributing to continued life is very unlikely.

(b) The preferences of the patient are not and cannot be known.

(c) The quality of life of the patient falls below the conditions that can, on the basis of widely held and reasonable criteria, be considered minimal.

(d) In the absence of current or prior patient preferences, appropriate surrogate decision-makers should be informed of the facts of the patient's condition, and the considerations noted above, and asked to agree to the abatement of continued life-support. Should surrogates refuse to agree, consult 2.8.

In cases where all these conditions are not fulfilled, poor quality of life should not be a decisive consideration. Indeed, it should be suspect; the sorts of judgments that healthy, intelligent, socially accomplished, and technically skilled persons make about the ill, incompetent, or uneducated and unskilled can often be biased. In addition, differences of social and economic class can lead to widely different views of what constitutes a tolerable quality of life. All sorts of "unacceptables" can be swept into the category of persons living "lives of poor quality" and thus not worthy of attention or care: addicts, the homeless, the uneducated and illiterate, persons of limited intelligence or with physical handicaps, those of unfamiliar cultural backgrounds, sexual preference or racial origins disfavored by the majority, and so on. Persons adjudged to fall into these vague categories may no longer be seen as "deserving help." This opens the way to invidious and destructive social policy and violates the ancient medical tradition that help be offered to all in need. Thus, quality-of-life considerations, although often relevant and on quite specific occasions decisive, should be viewed very cautiously when invoked to justify an ethical decision about whether medical treatment should be provided.

**3.5          EUTHANASIA AND ASSISTED SUICIDE**

Some persons may reach the conclusion that the quality of their life is so diminished that life is no longer worth living. This conclusion may be the result of unrelieved pain or suffering, or because they consider the prospect of deterioration, loss of spouse or friends unacceptable, or because they judge their lives to be a burden on others. Persons who come to this conclusion are sometimes terminally ill and under the care of a physician. They may request their physician to cause their death quickly and painlessly. In other cases, patients may be incapable of expressing such a desire to anyone, yet appear to be suffering so much that some other person, a friend, family member or care provider, may feel compelled to end their apparent suffering by causing their death. The term "euthanasia" has long been used to describe situations of both sorts. [EB: "Death and Dying: Euthanasia and Sustaining Life," I, 577–588; PBE, "Nonmaleficence," ch. 4; ME: Brock DW, "Death and Dying," 363–394; Beauchamp T, Veatch RM. *Ethical Issues in Death and Dying.* Upper Saddle River: Prentice-Hall, 1996; Legal Euthanasia: Ethical Issues in an Era of Legalized Aid-in-Dying. *J Med Philos* 1993; 18; Physician-Aided Death: The Escalating Debate. Special Section. *Cambridge Quarterly of Healthcare Ethics* 1996; 5 (1).]

### 3.5.1    Definition

The word "euthanasia," which literally means "good death," has been used in many different ways, resulting in considerable confusion. It was long used as a synonym for "mercy killing," that is, deliberately and directly killing a sufferer in order to relieve pain. More careful usage distinguished among "voluntary," "nonvoluntary," and "involuntary" euthanasia. Voluntary euthanasia describes situations in which the patient consciously and deliberately requested death. Nonvoluntary describes situations in which the patient was decisionally incapacitated and made no request. Involuntary describes situations in which the patients were killed against their wishes. These distinctions, while clarifying to some extent, also cause confusion. In recent years, involuntary euthanasia has been condemned by all commentators and nonvoluntary euthanasia, causing death without the expressed desire of the patient, has been condemned by most commentators. The debate now focuses on "voluntary euthanasia."

New terms have appeared in recent discussions. Various authors choose different terms to describe different situations. For the sake of clarity, we choose to use the phrase "aid-in-dying" to describe a situation in which a patient requests a physician to administer a lethal drug. We choose the phrase "physician-assisted suicide" to describe a death that a competent person deliberately chooses and also causes by self-administration of a substance which a physician prescribes but does not administer. Since the choice of the patient is central to both concepts, the ethics of both situations could have been discussed in Chapter 2, Preferences of Patients, but since the patient's choice is commonly associated, in legal and ethical discussions, with diminished quality of life, we choose to discuss it here.

**Case I.**    Mrs. Care is suffering from advanced MS. She is blind, bed-bound, obtunded, and appears to be in constant pain. Her husband asks the physician to end her suffering by ending her life. The physician administers a strong sedative, followed by an intravenous bolus of 120 millequivalents of potassium chloride.

**Case II.**    Ms. Comfort is dying from widely disseminated cancer and is suffering intense and implacable pain due to bony metastases, even though receiving high doses of morphine. She remains conscious and alert. She begs her doctor "to put her to sleep forever." The physician administers 200 mg of morphine sulfate intravenously.

**Case III.** Ms. Comfort is in the same situation as in Case II, but requests her physician to prescribe a supply of barbiturates sufficient for her to end her life, to give her and her husband instructions about appropriate dosage and administration and to be present when she herself takes the prescribed medication to end her life.

*COMMENT:* In all cases, the physician supplies a means that will rapidly and definitively interrupt an organic process that is necessary to continued life. This fact distinguishes these cases from the cases in 1.2, 2.5, and 3.2, where the physician stopped or did not provide some intervention for the support of failing vital processes. In Cases I and II, the physician acts directly to kill the patient. Not only does this not correspond to any currently recognized duty of physicians but also is contrary to law in all American jurisdictions. Case III presents the problem of physician-assisted suicide.

### 3.5.2 Physician-Assisted Suicide

Until recently, the exact nature of the physician's assistance in hastening death was not carefully defined. It was assumed that the physician would either prescribe or administer a lethal drug. In more recent discussions, the physician's role has been more precisely defined by those who advocate legalization of the physician's participation. Administration of a lethal drug presumably constitutes an act of homicide. However, prescription of drugs which the patient can take at will removes the physician from direct participation. The decision and the action of ending life remain in the patient's control. The patient, then, commits suicide, which is not an illegal act (3.6.3). The physician's participation by providing the means should, say advocates, be clearly excluded from statutes that prohibit aiding in suicide. Physician participation, these advocates claim, is in fact a proper medical duty of relief of pain. This description is called "physician-assisted suicide." It has increasingly become the favored way of presenting the issue. [Weir R, ed. *Physician Assisted Suicide.* Bloomington, Ind.: Indiana University Press, 1997; Physician-assisted suicide: Toward a comprehensive understanding. Report of the Task Force on Physician-Assisted

Suicide of the Society for Health and Human Values. *Academic Medicine,* 1995, 70:583–590; Special Section: Physician-Aided Death: The Escalating Debate. *Cambridge Quarterly of Healthcare Ethics* 1996, 6 (1).]

### 3.5.3    Ethical Arguments

The public, the medical community and medical ethicists are divided about the ethical propriety of physician-assisted suicide. The opponents of assisted suicide argue:

(a) Prohibition of the direct taking of human life, except in self-defense or in the defense of others, has been a central tenet of the Judeo-Christian tradition. It has been equally strong in the secular ethic. An ancient maxim of the Western legal tradition states that even the consent of the victim is not a defense against homicide.

(b) The ethics of medicine has traditionally emphasized the saving and preservation of life and the improvement of its quality and has repudiated the direct taking of life. The Hippocratic oath states: "I will not administer a deadly poison to anyone when asked to do so nor suggest such a course." Contemporary organized medicine reaffirms this tradition. The Council on Ethical and Judicial Affairs of the AMA states: "active euthanasia. . . is not a part of the practice of medicine with or without the consent of the patient." The American College of Physicians adds: "even if legalized, such an action would violate the ethical standards of medical practice." [AMA Council on Ethical and Judicial Affairs, *Current Opinions,* 1989; *American College of Physicians' Ethics Manual,* 2nd ed. Philadelphia: American College of Physicians, 1989.]

(c) The dedication of the medical profession to the welfare of patients and to the promotion of health might be seriously undermined in the eyes of the public and of patients by the complicity of physicians in the death of the very ill, even of those who request it. It is possible that subtle changes would enter into the relationship of patients and their physicians should such a practice become common.

(d) Requests for swift death are often made in circumstances of extreme distress which may be alleviated by skillful pain management and other positive interventions such as those employed in hospice care.

(e) Even if initial toleration of physician-assisted suicide is limited to the voluntary situation, it is possible that, once established, the practice might become more acceptable for involuntary patients who "would have requested" if they had been able. Similarly, the availability of quick death may bring subtle coercion on persons who feel that their invalid state is a burden to others. Thus, even when effecting a swift death at the request of a suffering patient seems merciful and benevolent, the acceptance of the practice as ethical may bear the seeds of frightening social consequences. The "euthanasia" program initiated in Germany in the first half of this century with the support of many benevolent physicians was first directed only to the incurably ill; it gradually expanded into genocide. This is the so-called slippery-slope argument (4.0.7).

Proponents of assisted suicide counter:

(a) The commonly invoked distinctions between "killing and allowing to die," "acting and refraining," etc., are spurious: thus, termination of treatment and direct killing are morally the same and, if the former is permitted, the latter should be also.

(b) Autonomous individuals have moral authority over their lives and should be allowed the means to end it, including the assistance of those who can do so painlessly and efficiently.

(c) No person should be coerced into bearing burdens of pain and suffering and those who relieve them of such burdens, at their request, are acting ethically, that is, out of compassion and respect for autonomy.

(d) Often the burdens of pain and disability are the result of the "success" of medical intervention to save life; those who have effected this result have an obligation to respect the patient's desire no longer to bear so unrewarding a result.

(e) The maxim of the Hippocratic oath is outdated, since medicine could never have anticipated the ability to extend dying as it has today. The maxim should be interpreted, as it is in the modern version, The Declaration of Geneva of the World Medical Association, "I will maintain the utmost respect for human life...."

(f) Some influential voices within the medical profession, which is generally opposed to active euthanasia, have recently expressed reasoned, carefully circumscribed support.

*COMMENT:*  These arguments pro and con are vigorously debated by proponents and opponents of assisted suicide. During the 1990s, efforts have been made, by legislation and by judicial decision, to make legal "physician-assisted suicide." In these efforts, legal considerations are added to ethical arguments. Even if legalization comes about, physicians will have to make conscientious decisions about whether to provide assistance to patients to end their lives. Also, even if legalized, the practice of physician-assisted suicide will require difficult decisions about what constitutes decisional capacity, terminal illness, and whether all means of relieving pain have been exhausted. In particular, the limited legal authorization—to competent patients in terminal illness—will leave questions about the patients in equally distressing circumstances who are unable to request or self-administer lethal medication and about persons who are not terminal but who anticipate slow death from degenerative disease.

A request for assistance in suicide should be met in the following manner:

(a) A physician who finds the arguments against assisting in suicide persuasive must inform the patient that he or she cannot in conscience cooperate, but then offer to discuss the issue in depth with the patient in hope of finding mutually acceptable options. If the patient continues to request assistance in suicide, the physician should offer to resign from the case.

(b) A physician who is persuaded by the arguments favoring assisted suicide must recognize that assisting in suicide is illegal (except in the state of Oregon at the time of this writing). Different jurisdictions have somewhat differing laws and different ways of dealing with the issue, but, in general, assisting suicide is a criminal act. A physician may choose to take the risk of legal liability, but should do so in full knowledge of the possible consequences.

(c) If a physician chooses to take the legal risk, he or she should be confident that the patient has decisional capacity and is suffering from a condition that can realistically be characterized as terminal. Consultation on these matters is advisable.

(d) The physician should explore the issue with the patient very carefully and sympathetically. The patient's medical situation, options for treatment, alternatives to suicide, comfort care, relief of pain, social supports, values, and attitudes should be discussed. The discussion should take place over time and might include others, such as the patient's spouse and children, closest friends, religious counselors, etc. A pattern for such a discussion is provided in Battin PM, "Rational suicide: how can we respond to a request for help?" *Crisis* 1991; 12:73–80.

*NOTE:* The phrase "death with dignity" is sometimes heard in discussions of allowing to die and causing death. We recommend against use of this phrase in serious ethical discussion. While appealing, the phrase is ambiguous and should not be allowed to carry weight in ethical deliberations without a precise definition of its meaning. If it is intended to mean that the expressed preferences of patients to refuse further medical intervention should be respected, "death with dignity" has important ethical significance: It is respect for the autonomy of the dying person. If it is intended to mean that dying persons should be spared the pain and inconvenience of repeated interventions of little utility, it also has ethical significance: It refers to the ethical obligation to shift from aggressive therapy to comforting care when therapy is futile. If the phrase is a defense of active, voluntary euthanasia or assisted suicide, it must be interpreted in light of the above reservations about this practice. Finally, if it is used to suggest that the suffering patient should be put "out of misery," it is ethically indefensible. The phrase "death with dignity" is most appropriately used to describe the obligation to care for the dying sensitively, compassionately, and ethically.

### 3.5.4 P  Infant Euthanasia

None of the arguments that favor physician-assisted suicide apply to infants or children. However, decisions to forgo life-sustaining treatment can be ethically justified. When such a decision is made, an infant or child may continue to live for a period of time and may experience what appears to be distress and pain. This raises the question whether it may be ethically permissible, even obligatory, to terminate the life of the infant immediately and directly, rather than tolerate a slow, painful death. Some authors see a compelling logic in this position. However, as a matter of practice, it is difficult to accept: the primary justification for euthanasia, namely, the voluntary consent of the patient, is absent; serious abuses might follow such toleration, and the killing of infants runs counter to the instincts of most persons. Adequate management of pain can be accomplished and measures of comfort instituted.

### 3.5.5  Legal Implications

Deliberately causing the death of another, unless justified or excused, constitutes a criminal act, as does cooperating in the causing of another's death. While suicide is not itself illegal,

nearly all the states have specific statutes against assisting someone to commit suicide. Thus, the physician who administers or
provides a lethal agent is liable to a criminal charge of homicide or
assisting suicide. Decisions to allow persons who are terminally
ill to die, discussed in the previous chapters and sections, are also
examples of "causing" the death of another. However, the clinical decision that further medical care would provide no therapeutic benefit other than to prolong organic life relieves the
physician of the legal duty to continue to intervene with medical
measures. Similarly, a competent patient has the right to have
life-supporting measures discontinued. These are clear and
accepted defenses against criminal and civil charges. A decision
to kill the patient by using some lethal agent, even when death
is imminent, does not rest on a clinical judgment about the futility of medical care. It is a decision that can be made by persons
without medical skills, and the lethal agent can be a bullet, an
electric shock, or poison. The "compassionate" intent of the per-
petrator is not a defense recognized by the law. Currently, the
request of the victim, even if competent and uncoerced, is not a
defense. In such situations, anyone who kills another human
being can be charged with a criminal offense. Physicians and
laypersons alike must stand before the law.

Three states (Washington, California, Oregon) have submitted
to their voters propositions to make legal the participation of
physicians in causing the death of competent, terminally ill persons who request them to do so. In Washington and California,
the proposition was narrowly defeated; in Oregon the voters
narrowly accepted this proposition which permitted "assisted
suicide" as defined above, although legal actions have prevented
the legislation from being put into effect. The United States
Supreme Court has ruled that state laws prohibiting assisted suicide are not unconstitutional, but that debate about its morality
and legality should continue, and it left open the possibility that
state law, such as Oregon's, might permit physician-assisted suicide in specified cases (Washington v. Glucksberg; Vacco v.
Quill; U.S. Sup Ct, 1997).

**3.6**                        **SUICIDE**

Suicide is the deliberate taking of one's life. It is natural to assume
that attempted or requested suicide in part reflects a personal
belief that the quality of one's life has become unbearable. As an

ethical problem, it could be discussed under patient preferences, Chapter 2. However, since the physician will often encounter the problem either at the end of the terminal illness of a patient, when life is of "poor quality," or in the emergency department, when preferences can only be inferred, it is discussed here. [EB: "Suicide," IV, 2444–2450; Battin MP, Mayo DJ, eds. *Suicide: The Philosophical Issues.* New York: St. Martin's Press, 1980.]

### 3.6.1    Treatment of Suspected Suicides

Suspected suicides are frequently encountered in the emergency room Even when the suspicion is supported by evidence, such as a history and a suicide note, it has been customary to provide all means necessary for resuscitation and care, if there are solid medical grounds to expect recovery.

**Case.**    Ms. D.W., a 24-year-old woman, is brought to the ER; she has deeply slashed her wrists and overdosed. She is obtunded. She has been brought in several times before and is known to have a psychiatric history of depression. On her last admission she screamed that next time she should be allowed to die.

*RECOMMENDATION:*    Ms. D.W. should be treated. The customary practice of disregarding the suicide wish in the emergency room situation is ethically appropriate, even though it seems to contravene the autonomy of the person.

(a) The ethical basis for suicide prevention is the well-authenticated psychological thesis that the suicide attempt is very often a "cry for help" rather than an unambivalent decision to end one's life. Frequently the very fact that the attempted suicide arrives in the ER suggests the act was ambivalently motivated. Many suicide attempts are halfway. The suicide attempt may not be an act of autonomy but rather be an act resulting from impaired capacity due to psychopathology or emotional conflict.

(b) Suicide attempts are often undertaken in psychopathological conditions which are treatable or under social conditions that are transient. It is sometimes possible to anticipate these problems. Physicians have an ethical obligation to recognize the suicidal inclinations of patients whom they encounter in their practice and to make efforts to assist them personally or by referral to a trained counselor.

### 3.6.2    Suicide and Refusal of Treatment

It is sometime asked whether refusal of treatment by a patient is equivalent to suicide. If it were, the physician might feel constrained to prevent suicide or to avoid complicity. There are significant ethical differences between suicide and refusal of medical care.

(a) In refusal of care, persons do not take their lives; rather they do not permit another to help them survive. Persons who abhor the thought of suicide may say, "I do not want to kill myself. I only want to be allowed to die."

(b) In refusal of care, death is caused by the progress of a lethal disease which is not treated; in suicide the immediate cause of death is a self-inflicted lethal act. In refusing lifesaving care the patient does not set in motion the lethal cause. The patient's refusal authorizes the physician to refrain from therapy; the fatal condition is itself the cause of death.

(c) Even though suicide and refusal of treatment both result in death, the moral setting differs completely in intention, circumstances, motives, and desires.

(d) The Roman Catholic Church, which condemns suicide, does permit its adherents to refuse care, even should death result, when treatment offers little hope and is burdensome, painful, or costly ("extraordinary").

(e) Many judicial decisions and legal statutes now distinguish between legitimate refusal of care and suicide. Most Natural Death Acts explicitly state that death following a decision authorized by these acts cannot be considered suicide for purposes of denial of life insurance.

### 3.6.3    Legal Status of Suicide

Suicide was a crime in the Anglo-American common law, but all sanctions for suicide (which formerly had included confiscation of the suicide's estate) were repealed in American jurisdictions in the first half of the twentieth century. Most jurisdictions retain legal sanctions against aiding and abetting suicides. These presumably apply to anyone who, under current law, provided aid-in-dying or physician-assisted suicide. Efforts are being made to revise these laws by making exceptions for physician participation in the suicide of terminally ill patients.

**3.7**                            **SUMMARY**

Quality of life describes both certain facts about a person's life and the value that person and others place on those facts. It is a pervasive concept in medical decision-making, yet it must be employed with care. It is open to serious bias and discrimination. It may be an important and sometimes a decisive consideration in deliberating about the appropriateness of forgoing life-support. Seriously diminished quality of life is offered as a rationale for euthanasia, but unless the patient personally requests assistance in dying, that rationale is not persuasive; even if the patient does make such a request, ethical controversy persists about assisted suicide, and law still prohibits it.

# CHAPTER 4

# Contextual Features

**4.0** This chapter reviews the fourth topic that is essential to the adequate description and resolution of a case in clinical ethics: the social, legal, and economic and institutional circumstances in which a particular case of patient care takes place. These circumstances are the context of the case and so we call the topic "contextual features." Physicians and patients have various responsibilities and obligations to the larger world in which their relationship takes place: they have families, live in social and political communities, and are employed by, or contract with, health care organizations. What is the import of varied responsibilities on the relationship between patient and physician?

Recent changes in the organization and delivery of health care force a close consideration of this question. The patient-physician encounter takes place in more complex institutional and economic structures than ever before. Only occasionally does the traditional private relationship exist in which a patient chooses and consults a physician for diagnosis and treatment, is given an evaluation and recommendation, and pays a fee for service. More often doctors today stand in multiple relationships with other physicians, nurses and allied health professionals, health care administrators, third-party payers, professional organizations, state and federal agencies, in addition to patients and their families. Similarly, patients stand in relationships with family and friends, other health professionals, health care institutions, and third-party payers. Not only is the traditional patient-physician relationship embedded in these multiple relationships, but physicians and patients are subject to the varying influence of multiple values—patients' preferences, physicians' goals, community and professional standards, legal rules, hospital policies, research regulations, teaching concerns, economic considerations, religious beliefs, and other factors. Further complicating factors include changes in health care financing, legal changes to reform health care access and delivery, and computerized medical information, storage, and retrieval. Contextual factors such as costs and reorganization of health care in particular have created conflicts of interest for physicians, who, in addition to serving their patient's needs, are increasingly called upon to take responsibility for utilization and costs of health care. This social burden often is, or is perceived to be, imposed at the expense of benefits to particular patients.

The context of care has assumed more prominence than ever before and influences the ways in which ethical problems are viewed, analyzed, and resolved. The context of care is related to the particular case in at least two ways: it establishes the limits and conditions in which decisions take place, and it is itself influenced by decisions made by and about the patient. For example, the economic context might be one in which a patient's insurance coverage is inadequate: this raises the ethical question for providers about whether to engage in costly interventions for that patient. In this chapter, we will discuss the ethical relevance of both of these aspects of the contextual features. Under the topic of contextual features, we discuss (1) the role of interested parties other than the patient, such as the patient's relatives, (2) the economics of medical care, (3) the allocation of medical resources, (4) the role of the law, (5) medical research and teaching, (6) safety and welfare of society.

### 4.0.1    Clinical Decisions and Policy Decisions

In this book, contextual features are discussed only in relation to clinical cases. These issues can also be discussed in terms of social, economic, and health policy. These policy discussions concern "macro-issues," that is, the overall construction of policies and institutions that affect large populations. This chapter is primarily limited to "micro-issues," that is, the relationship between the contextual features and the care of the individual patient.

*EXAMPLE:*    Mr. Cope, the diabetic patient in 2.2.2 and 2.9, is now hospitalized for treatment of severe ketoacidosis. Ulcerations on his legs are not healing. He has continued to be noncompliant and his alcohol abuse has become severe. His renal function has deteriorated gradually and he now has end-stage renal disease. The question of dialysis is raised. Mr. Cope's primary care physician advises against it on the grounds that the patient's history of poor compliance with medical regimens makes him a poor candidate. The nephrologist comments that, since the End-Stage Renal Disease Program pays for the treatment, it is worth a try. The primary care physician states that this might be an opportunity to save the End-Stage Renal Disease program some money.

*COMMENT:* The costs of chronic hemodialysis are paid by a federal program, the End-Stage Renal Disease Program. This program is thought by some to be disproportionately expensive relative to the number of patients served. A question of justice might be raised about how to develop a policy that would restrain costs and ration the service. This is a problem distinct from the clinical problem of deciding whether Mr. Cope ought to go on dialysis. Although governmental and institutional policies are relevant to clinical cases, their ethical aspects as policies that promote or hinder just and fair allocation of care is not directly discussed in our pages.

*RECOMMENDATION:* The decision about putting Mr. Cope on dialysis should be made above all on the basis of medical indications, patient preferences, and quality of life. Since Mr. Cope has not been cooperative with medical treatment, the primary care physician's first recommendation deserves some consideration. His suggestion about saving the ESRD program some money is not directly relevant to this clinical decision.

## 4.0.2  Justice and Public Policies

Many ethical problems in clinical decisions are caused by public policies and the structures of institutions. For a variety of reasons, such as limited fiscal resources, political pressures, or legal provisions, decisions about patients may be constrained or limited in ways that inhibit the care of the patient in ways that seem ethically inappropriate. Individual physicians and patients may be able to do little about these circumstances. Thus, they may be faced with undesirable options for ethical choice. Although we are vividly aware that inequitable, inefficient, or inadequate social policies do create situations where all ethical options are

less than ideal, this chapter does not propose the reforms of
social policy that may be desirable. However, physicians should
be involved in the development of social policies and their
application to patient care. Justice, the ethics of fair and equitable distribution of burdens and benefits within a community,
is often the most relevant ethical principle for the formulation
and application of social policy. Classically defined as "giving to
each his due," different theories of justice debate about what is
"due" and to whom it is due. In general, the maxims, "to each
equally," "to each according to contribution," "to each according
to merit," "to each according to need," compete for priority. In
health care, the criterion of need is often the determining one
for distribution of medical services, yet even in the application
of this criterion, problems arise. These problems will be noted
below, particularly in discussing the allocation of scarce resources: [EB: "Justice," II, 1308–1318, "Health Care Resources,
Allocation of," II, 1067–1083; PBE: "Justice," ch. 6, 326–386;
ME: Daniels N. "National Health Care Reform," ch. 14, 415–442;
Daniels N. *Just Health Care*. Cambridge: Cambridge University
Press, 1985; Churchill L. *Self-Interest and Universal Health Care*.
Cambridge: Harvard University Press, 1994; Daniels N. *Seeking
Fair Treatment: From the AIDS Epidemic to National Health
Care Reform*. New York: Oxford University Press, 1995; Can
Justice Endure Health Care Reform? Special Section. *Cambridge
Quarterly of Healthcare Ethics*. 1996; 5(4).]

### 4.0.3    Loyalty and the Multiple Responsibilities of Physicians

The ethics of medicine has traditionally directed the physician to
attend primarily, even exclusively, to the needs of the patient. It
is clearly unethical to do anything to a patient that will not benefit, and may even harm, the patient in order to benefit the
physician or some other party. For example, a physician who
performs diagnostic or therapeutic procedures that are not indicated, under pretense of caring for the patient but with the
intent only of collecting a Medicaid fee, clearly acts unethically.
At the same time, it has always been recognized that physicians,
in some sense, also have certain responsibilities beyond their
patients. The Preamble of the Principles of Medical Ethics of the
AMA expresses this: "The medical profession has long sub-
scribed to a body of ethical statements developed primarily for
the benefit of the patient. As a member of this profession, a

physician must recognize the responsibility not only to patients, but also to society, to other health professionals, and to self" (AMA Principles, 1957). In recent years, the absorption of the once very private relationship between physicians and patients into large organizations which employ or contract with physicians and which enroll and insure patients has added a new dimension to the physician's duties. Frequently, physicians take on contractual obligations with these organizations which directly affect the ways in which they care for their patients.

The ethical problem posed by multiple responsibilities arises when it is unclear how to determine which responsibilities have priority in a particular case or when it appears that duty to one's patient are in direct conflict with duties to others. The moral principle of loyalty is appropriate to these problems. Loyalty is a sustained commitment to the welfare of persons or to the success of an endeavor, requiring an investment of effort and sometimes even a subordination of self-interest. All persons have multiple loyalties—to family, to friends, to a religious faith, to a community, a nation, a cause—and usually these can be managed without conflict. At times, different loyalties will draw a person in divergent directions, between which a choice must be made. The tradition of medical ethics, the expectation of the public, and the common law assign a high priority to the physician's loyalty to his or her patients; we will discuss the conditions which limit that loyalty in the following sections. [EB: "Fidelity and Loyalty," II, 864–868; PBE: "Patient-Physician Relationships," ch. 7, 395–462; Ramsey P. *The Patient as Person.* New Haven: Yale University Press, 1970; Toulmin, SE. Divided loyalties and ambiguous relationships. *Soc Sci Med* 1986; 23:784.]

### 4.0.4 Fiduciary Duty

It is often said that physicians have, under law, a fiduciary duty to their patients. A fiduciary owes undivided loyalty to those served and must work for their benefit. Fiduciaries have specialized expertise and are held to high standards of honesty, confidentiality, and loyalty. Above all, fiduciaries must avoid financial conflict of interest that could prejudice their clients' interests. Thus, physicians, lawyers, accountants, engineers, and architects are typically considered fiduciaries, from whom clients are entitled to expect such performance and may sue if they are disappointed.

Despite the fiduciary rhetoric, the concept is clouded in practice. Courts and legislatures tailor the fiduciary metaphor to meet the nuances of particular cases and patterns of social responsibilities. Law applies the concept to medicine principally in contexts of abandonment, confidentiality, informed consent, and disclosure of financial interests. Some economic conflicts are prohibited, but many exceptions exist. Neither malpractice law nor licensing rules invoke fiduciary standards. Many new contractual and organizational arrangements in health care put great strain on a concept that has limited applicability. Merely invoking the fiduciary nature of the relationship does not solve the ethical and legal problems posed by the new context of health care.

### 4.0.5 Conflict of Interest

The term "conflict of interest" is often used to describe a situation in which a person might be motivated to perform actions that his or her professional role makes possible but which are at variance with the acknowledged duties of that role. The term applies most clearly to persons who hold political office and who can use the powers of office to enrich themselves. More recently, the concept has been applied to other professions, including medicine. [EB: "Conflict of Interest," I, 459–464; *Current Opinions of AMA*. Conflicts of Interest, 8.03–8.035; Spece RG, Shimm DS, Buchanan AE. *Conflicts of Interest in Clinical Practice and Research*. New York: Oxford University Press, 1996; Rodwin MA. *Medicine, Money and Morals*. New York: Oxford University Press, 1993; Symposium on conflict of interest in health care. *Am J Law Med* 1995; 21 (2 & 3).]

*EXAMPLE:* A group of internists pool resources to invest in an imaging facility. The volume of business at that facility creates profits for them. The prospect of profit may influence their clinical judgments about the need for various diagnostic imaging for their patients.

*EXAMPLE:* A pharmaceutical company recruits a number of cardiologists in private practice to perform clinical studies of the antihypertensive effects of a new calcium channel blocker. The company pays physicians a bonus for each patient who completes the study. The utilization review team discovers a substantial decline in the cardiologists' use of ACE inhibitors and of the calcium channel blockers listed in the group's formulary.

*EXAMPLE:* A managed care organization recruits physicians by offering a generous incentive program in which physicians can receive a bonus of up to 50 percent of their base salary depending on their record of not using high-cost medical interventions, including hospitalization, to care for a group of capitated patients.

*COMMENT:* A conflict of interest is not in itself unethical. It is a situation in which an individual is provided the opportunity and motivation to act contrary to duty in order to gain personal benefit. Some conflicts of interest can be avoided, e.g., by a law that would forbid physicians to own centers for self-referral, or by creating a presumption that such a situation is suspect, e.g., the AMA declaration that it is unethical for physicians to own centers for self-referral unless this is the only way to meet a special community need. [AMA Council on Ethical and Judicial Affairs. Conflicts of interest: physicians ownership of medical facilities. *JAMA* 1992; 267: 2366–2369, *Current Opinions,* 8.032.] It is also generally recommended that those who are in a conflict of interest declare this conflict openly to those who may be affected by it. However, in the complex setting of contemporary health care, many conflicts of interest are subtle.

## 4.0.6    Relevance of Contextual Features

Many physicians feel strongly that they have a primary duty to their particular patients. This is as it should be. However, a primary duty is neither absolute nor exclusive of other duties. It is, as we noted above, conditioned by moral obligations arising from justice and loyalty, which on occasion will require favoring the rights and welfare of parties other than their particular patients. This is so for several reasons:

(a) Professional ethics, even though they place special demands on physicians toward their patients, do not exempt them from general ethical obligations incumbent upon all. Obligations of justice are of such a nature.

(b) The professions themselves exist and enjoy a privileged position because society expects them to serve the public welfare. Professional commitment to particular individuals is encouraged and tolerated up to the point where it might endanger the public health or safety.

(c) Patients and physicians are often participants in cooperative arrangements, such as insurance plans or health maintenance organizations, which establish reciprocal relationships to other members of such arrangements. Physician advocacy of the welfare of their individual patients is modified by the just contractual conditions of such arrangements.

*COMMENT:* While duty to the patient, based on medical indications, patient preferences, and quality of life, will usually constitute the primary feature to be considered in ethical decisions in clinical care, on occasion, contextual features will loom large and sometimes will be decisive. Given the multiplicity and complexity of these features, it is difficult to state any general rule about the priority of contextual features. As a general principle, we propose that contextual features should not be decisive over consideration of (1) medical indications, (2) patient preference, and (3) quality of life. However, contextual features become more decisive in clinical decisions when all of the following conditions are met:

(a) The achievement of significant goals of medical intervention is doubtful.

(b) The preferences of the patient are not and cannot be known.

(c) The quality of the patient's life is minimal or below minimal.

(d) The contextual feature in question is specific, notably burdensome to others, and the decision will make a difference in alleviating that burden.

### 4.0.7    Slippery-Slope Arguments

The claim that toleration of a certain action or policy as ethical will lead to unwanted consequences is often heard. Since, in medical ethics, those unwanted consequences often fall into the category of contextual features, we mention the "slippery-slope arguments" here. In these arguments, the original act or policy proposed does not seem to contravene any ethical principle and so, apart from the unwanted consequences, would be ethically acceptable. For example, it might be argued that assisted suicide does not contravene the principle of respect for autonomy, nor the principle of beneficence and nonmaleficence; however, its toleration will lead to widespread disregard for the lives of the disabled. Slippery-slope arguments are built on the premise that acceptance of some act or policy is contagious because persons are psychologically inclined to move from one step to the next, or from narrow to wider interpretations. This form of argument is not, in itself, persuasive, since it contains many assumptions difficult to prove, but it does urge a closer, more thoughtful examination of the issue.

## 4.1          ROLE OF INTERESTED PARTIES

Physicians have a moral and legal obligation to exercise special care to promote the interests of their patients. Patients have an interest in the competence and honesty of their physicians and an interest in the appropriate response to their health needs. Thus, the primary interested parties in a clinical encounter are the patient and the physician. However, many other parties may have some interest in that encounter and its outcome. Traditionally, families have such an interest, and physicians have recognized the legitimacy of that interest. The authority of the family to participate in decisions about their relative's care is explained in 2.7. In modern medical care, many other parties claim interest in the care of patients: hospital and managed care administrators, public health authorities, third-party payers, employers, litigants, lawyers, etc. They may seek information, exercise oversight, establish policies that affect care decisions, and even attempt to dictate care. The justification of the legitimacy of these various claims is the ethical issue.

### 4.1.1   Allegiance and Advocacy

Physicians owe allegiance to their patients, that is, they must respect their patients' preferences and privacy and respond to their health and informational needs. This allegiance is an expression of loyalty. This allegiance requires that physicians advocate their patients' interests, such as access to the most appropriate care or the preservation of confidential information, before the interests of parties outside the primary relationship. However, this allegiance, while a strong obligation, is not absolute, nor is the stringent duty of advocacy unlimited. The special obligations of professional ethics do not exempt physicians from general moral obligations. The exceptions to allegiance and the limits of justice are set by the ethically justified claims of other parties. We shall develop this point in each of the subsequent Contextual Features.

### 4.1.2   Physician's Duty to Self and Family

Every physician, like every human being, has certain moral duties to self and to those who constitute immediate family, such as spouse and children. Duties to self include adherence to one's values, cultivation of one's talents, preservation of health; duties to family include specially stringent obligations to promote their welfare and protect them from harm. There may be situations when physicians are faced with performances of duties toward their patients that entail risk to themselves and, indirectly, to their family.

**Case.**    Dr. O., a 36-year-old orthopedic surgeon in private practice, instructs his office staff to "screen" prospective patients, noting any characteristics that suggest they might be in a high-risk group for HIV infection. They are to inform such persons that Dr. O. is unable to accept new patients at this time. He also has an ELISA test performed on all patients without their knowledge. He defends his actions by asserting his right, and the right of his wife and any future child, to protection from infection.

*COMMENT:*    The duty to preserve health and protect family, with the corresponding right to do so, is legitimate, but it must be evaluated in terms of the nature, probability, and seriousness of the risks, alternative strategies, the infringement on others' rights, and the social consequences of various courses of action. In this matter:

(a) For health professionals in general, the danger of infection by contact with a patient is low, but not negligible. The risks for orthopedic surgeons, given the nature of their work, is probably somewhat greater than for other surgeons and considerably greater than for physicians who do not have regular contact with bodily fluids. Risk of infection is related to the potential for percutaneous exposure to blood. Hollow-bore needle sticks pose the greatest risk to health professionals, and thus nurses, phlebotomists, house officers, and medical students are the groups at greatest risk. After a hollow-bore needle stick, risk of HIV infection appears to be very low—about 0.3 percent overall. Further postexposure prophylaxis with AZT effectively reduces the transmission rate, by 79 percent according to one study. [CDC case control study of HIV seroconversion in health care workers after percutaneous exposure to HIV infected blood. *MMWR* 1995; 44:929–933.]

(b) Various protective procedures have been devised that, if properly used, appear to be an effective barrier to infection.

(c) Medical tradition praises those who care for patients at risk to themselves. Medicine's public reputation rests in part on this tradition, and the public expects physicians to act in this way, so far as is reasonable.

(d) Toleration of the practice of excluding HIV-positive patients would lead to the exclusion of many persons in serious need of care and the exclusion of many who are incorrectly identified as infected.

(e) All major medical organizations have asserted the obligation of physicians to treat patients with HIV infection. The AMA Ethical and Judicial Council states, "A physician may not ethically refuse to treat a patient whose condition is within the physician's realm of competence ... neither those who have the disease (AIDS) nor those who have been infected with the virus should be subject to discrimination based on fear or prejudice, least of all by members of the health care community." [AMA Ethical and Judicial Council Opinion 9.131, Council Report. Ethical issues in the growing AIDS crisis. *JAMA* 1988; 259: 1360–1361.]

(f) In Dr. O.'s case, he is using methods that are inappropriate, inefficient, and unethical. The "screen" depends on stereotypes and will not efficiently exclude infected patients. HIV testing without consent is clearly unethical and, in many jurisdictions, illegal. It is not inappropriate, however, to urge voluntary testing in patients who might pose risks. [ME: Bayer R, "AIDS and Ethics," ch. 13, 395–413.]

### 4.1.3 Family, Relatives and Friends

Patients are located in a social context of other persons with whom they have various sorts of relationships and interaction. These others are often interested in the medical problems of the patient and sometimes play an important role in the way care is provided. Their role as surrogate decision-makers is discussed in 2.7. They may have other roles, such as providing emotional or living support, providing information, serving as interpreter of the patient's values, paying the bills. They may sometimes engage in controversy about the course of care and seek to serve their own interests rather than the patient's. The moral cooperation of these others should be sought and encouraged; their moral roles and claims must occasionally be sorted out. In Chapter 2 we discussed the issues surrounding cultural differences. Role of families is often defined quite differently in other cultures, and ethical problems will sometimes arise

**Case.** A Japanese-American family brings their maternal grandmother to their primary care physician. Grandmother is 72 years old, came to the United States ten years ago, and speaks no English. She complains of weakness, weight loss, nausea, and fever of several months duration. Her son, who is a computer engineer, tells the doctor "in case you find cancer, we prefer that she not be told. That is the way with our older people. But we do want her to have full treatment." Studies reveal acute lymphocytic leukemia (ALL) with renal failure, a condition which has a 5 percent chance for clinical response to aggressive and prolonged chemotherapy.

*RECOMMENDATION:* In Chapter 2 we stated our repudiation of paternalism and, at the same time, our wish to respect, as far as possible, cultural values. In this case, we recommend that the patient be informed, through a reliable translator, that she is very sick, that decisions must be made about her care, and then asked whether she wishes to make these decisions for herself or prefers to have them made by another. An authorized delegation of decisional authority rather than simply accepting the culture's customs is an appropriate compromise.

### 4.1.4 P  The Family

In pediatrics, families are of central importance. The authority of parents as decision-makers in the care of a sick child is discussed in 2.7.5 P. The primary responsibility of parents must be the welfare of their child. However, the parents of an ill child are often parents of other children and have multiple responsibilities. Decisions about treatment may have major implications for their other children and for the social and financial stability of the family. Often, parents will devote almost exclusive attention to the sick child but, on occasion they ask themselves whether this is unfair to themselves and their other children. [EB: "Family," II, 801–807; Meyers DT, Kipnis K, Murphy CF. *Kindred Matters. Rethinking the Philosophy of the Family.* Ithaca: Cornell University Press, 1993.]

**Case.** In 3.0.10 P, we have seen Monica, born with a major myelodysplasia. Her parents have three other children, 12, 8, and 4 years of age. The 8-year-old also has a neural tube defect of lesser severity but is hydrocephalic with a shunt and is somewhat retarded. The family gains its livelihood on a small, unproductive farm and lives at some distance from schools and medical facilities. They have been very devoted to the care and education of the 8-year-old and are fearful that the other two children are suffering from the attention given her. They now face the prospect of another handicapped child.

*COMMENT:* In the case at 3.0.10 P, we recommended that medical intervention for Monica could be omitted, in accord with the parents' wishes. However, that counsel was offered in view of the prospects of a life of great pain and suffering for the patient. The welfare of this family and of the other children was not, in itself, the primary justification. Nevertheless, it is an additional consideration that, while not in itself decisive, deserves attention and may become decisive.

### 4.1.5 P  Providers' View of Family

In 2.7.7 P, the problem of incompetent parents was noted. Physicians and nurses caring for the sick infant or child may form views of a family that affect their attitude toward treatment. A family of different cultural background or socioeconomic status than providers are accustomed to dealing with may bias them against taking the parents' wishes seriously. On occasion, the perceived problems may be very real—for example, when both mother and father are addicted to drugs and alcohol, live in substandard conditions, and so forth. In other cases, the perception might be quite inaccurate. For example, Monica's parents were "mountain people," whose life-style and appearance were quite foreign to the staff of the distant medical center. Yet, they were caring and competent parents who made great sacrifices for their children. Again, appearances may deceive in the other direction. Intelligent and achieving parents, in protecting their social and economic status, may act to the detriment of their child's best interests and, because of their appearance and manner, be tolerated by providers. Cultural customs, such as the Laotian practice of placing heated coins on a sick baby's body, may appear to providers as child abuse. When faced with such situations, providers must first ask themselves whether their judgments are affected by their own biases and ignorance. If problems are genuine and pose a threat to the infant or child in the home environment, educational means should be employed and, if they fail, legal action initiated through the child protective agency.

4.2					**CONFIDENTIALITY**

Other parties are sometimes interested in the sensitive personal information that a patient discloses to a physician. That information is traditionally, ethically, and legally guarded by confidentiality. Physicians are obliged to refrain from divulging information obtained from patients and to take reasonable precautions to assure that such information is not inappropriately divulged by others to whom it might be professionally known. The duty of medical confidentiality is an ancient one: the Hippocratic oath states, "what I may see or hear in or outside the course of treatment ... which on no account must be spread abroad, I will keep to myself, holding such things shameful to speak about." Modern medical ethics bases this duty on respect for the autonomy of the patient, on the fidelity owed by the physician, and on the possibility that disregard of confidentiality would discourage patients from revealing useful diagnostic information and encourage others to use medical information to exploit patients. Confidentiality is a stringent, but not an absolute, obligation. The ethical issue, then, is determining what principles and circumstances justify exception to the rule. This is perhaps one of the most difficult problems in medical ethics: the value of confidentiality requires that the physician who considers breaching it have the most serious justification. The ethical justifications for breaching confidentiality are based on the principle of justice and depend upon the contextual features of the case. In general, two grounds for exception exist: concern for the safety of other specific persons and concern for public welfare. Both involve the possibility that other parties will be unjustly harmed.

Confidentiality may be treated rather carelessly in modern medical care. Providers may speak about patients in public places. Records are not well secured and are accessible to many persons, including some who are not health professionals. The greatest challenge to confidentiality in modern medical care results from technological developments in information storage, retrieval, and access. Computerization of medical records enhances statistical information and facilitates administrative tasks. But the availability of medical record information to interested third parties—employers, government agencies, payers, family members, and others—threatens patient or even physician control over sensitive information. For example, growing use of screening for genetic diseases, or susceptibility to them, produces information of interest, not only to patients and their physicians, but to the patient's relatives, employers, and insurers. Lack of consensus about how to regulate access to such information poses a continuing problem for health care institutions and policy-makers. Legal protection of confidentiality is uneven, with variable state laws and no comprehensive federal legislation defining the value, scope, or limits of confidentiality. Physicians, then, who bear the responsibility to protect their patient's confidentiality, must be as vigilant as possible and must advocate for better control of information and for better policy and law to safeguard it. [EB: "Confidentiality," I, 451–458; PBE: ch. 7, "Professional-Patient Relationships," 418–428; ME: Brody H. "The Physician-Patient Relationship," ch. 4, 89–92.]

## 4.2.1 Confidentiality and the Safety of Individuals

Confidential information may be divulged to appropriate persons when a physician is aware that lack of that information places some identifiable person at high risk of serious harm.

**Case I.** A 61-year-old man is diagnosed with metastatic cancer of the prostate. He refuses hormonal therapy and chemotherapy. He commands his physician not to inform his wife and says he does not intend to tell her himself. The next day, the wife calls to inquire about her husband's health.

**Case II.** A 32-year-old man is diagnosed presymptomatically with Huntington's disease. This is an autosomal dominant genetic disease (50 percent chance of transmitting the gene, and the disease, to offspring). He tells his physician that he does not want his wife, whom he has recently married, to know. The physician knows that the wife is eager to have children.

**Case III.** A 27-year-old gay man is diagnosed as HIV-positive. He tells his physician that he cannot face the prospect that his lover will learn of the infection.

*RECOMMENDATION:* In Case I, the physician should not divulge the husband's diagnosis. While the wife has a moral right to know of her husband's condition, which will certainly affect her deeply, it is her husband's obligation to inform her. The physician, while feeling distressed about the situation, cannot justify disclosure because his obligation to respect his patient's preferences outweighs possible harm to the wife from not knowing her husband's diagnosis. The physician should encourage the husband to reveal his condition but should not himself divulge the diagnosis to his wife. In Case II, there is a stronger rationale for divulging the diagnosis to the patient's wife. However, serious efforts should be made to convince the husband to seek genetic counseling and to urge him to discuss the matter with his wife. If the wife is also a patient, the physician may encourage her to talk seriously with her husband about his health and their plans for children. Risk of harm to future children is high (50 percent), but that risk is statistical and might not eventuate. There is no assurance that the breach of confidentiality will protect any given individual. Still, the risk of harm to the marriage and, possibly, to future children favors disclosure as a last resort. In Case III, the physician has a duty to assure that the lover is informed of his serious risk, first by urging the patient to do so and, if this is unavailing, by taking the steps prescribed in public health law and practice to assure that the person at risk is notified.

## 4.2.2    Legal Implications

In a precedent-setting case, Tarasoff v. Regents (Cal. Sup. Ct., 1976), a student informed his psychotherapist that he intended to kill a young woman. This was not communicated to the woman, whom the student subsequently murdered. The court ruled that the psychotherapist had a positive duty to take reasonable steps to protect third parties from harm, stating "the protective privilege (of confidentiality) ends where the public peril begins." The serious danger of violence to an identifiable person was a consideration that, in the opinion of the court, overrode the obligation to preserve confidential information obtained in the course of therapy. It is unclear how this decision would apply to other practitioners who obtain similar information in the course of providing general medical care. In recent years, this decision has provided a model for the advice given that counsels physicians to inform specific persons at risk of HIV infection. It is important, however, that any physician who does so be certain of the identity of the persons involved, of the high probability of risk, and make use of any established public health means of contact tracing.

## 4.2.3    Confidentiality and Public Welfare

Certain information obtained from patients may suggest that the patient might endanger others but without being able to identify specific others or occasions. Traditionally, certain communicable diseases have belonged in this category, and laws have been enacted that require physicians to report cases of communicable disease to health authorities. Many jurisdictions require reporting of health defects, such as seizures and cardiac pathologies, that might render operators of vehicles dangerous to others. Where reporting laws do not exist, and often even when they do, ethical problems may arise.

**Case I.**    Mr. Cure, with bacterial meningitis (probably pneumococcal but possibly meningococcal), refuses therapy and insists on returning to his college dormitory room.

**Case II.**    A 28-year-old man who has been under a physician's care for severe peptic ulcer impresses his doctor as somewhat bizarre in attitude and behavior. He suspects that his patient suffers from a psychotic disorder and asks him whether he is seeing a psychiatrist. He calmly responds that he was once under treatment for schizophrenia but has been well for years. Then, in the course of an office visit, he casually states that he would like to see all politicians dead and was going to attend a forthcoming political rally "to see what he could do." Should the physician report the patient to the police?

**Case III.**    A 27-year-old nurse in a dialysis unit is hepatitis B antigen-positive. She is reluctant to inform her social contacts and resists any restriction of her professional activities. She approaches a private practitioner for advice. She insists on confidentiality and after being advised to tell the relevant parties, including the hospital's infection control team, states that she does not intend to do so. Should the practitioner take steps to ensure that her social contacts are informed? Should the practitioner take steps to have her professional activities restricted?

**Case IV.** A school board considers a policy of requiring HIV antibody tests for all teachers. The results of the test would be available to the board. The board asks its physician for advice.

*COMMENT:* In Case I, bacterial meningitis is an infectious disease. If it is listed as a reportable communicable disease, the physician should report it. Since the final diagnosis is not clear and could be meningococcal meningitis, which is contagious, the physician has the duty to communicate the information to college authorities and recommend that Mr. Cure be isolated in the college infirmary during the course of his illness. In Case II, the danger to others is less clear. This patient is obviously in need of psychiatric treatment and should be persuaded to seek it. The threat is vague and, as is often the case, possibly empty. The conditions mentioned in 4.2.2 are absent: no victim is identified and the likelihood of violence is uncertain. The consequences to the patient of a police report might be significant. The consequences of reporting "suspicious persons" on the basis of suspicions aroused in medical care might also be socially undesirable.

In Case III, the nurse may infect others and the possibilities for contact are extensive and difficult to limit. She is capable of arranging her social contacts so as to avoid infecting others. In terms of her professional life, she has a direct obligation to protect her patients from harm. If she refuses to do this by reporting herself and by restricting her activities voluntarily, the physician has a duty to report her to the hospital authorities. In Case IV, the HIV antibody test in a population without risk factors for AIDS yields a high percentage of false positives, and even if some teachers are truly seropositive, their work does not entail activities that are associated with infectivity. The physician should strongly advise against the policy and provide the scientific reasons why it is inadvisable. In many states, a policy such as this would violate state laws regarding confidentiality of HIV status.

*RECOMMENDATION:* The ethical obligation to protect others, even at the expense of interfering with the patient's liberty and privacy, is strongest in Case I. There is a genuine threat of serious harm to other persons. In Case II, we do not consider the eventuality of harm sufficiently likely to justify a breach of confidentiality, although more information may heighten assurance that the patient is very likely to act out his fantasies. A threat to a particular person should be reported. In Case III, the more remote risk, the responsibility of the person for her own behavior and the practical impossibility of protecting everyone with whom she deals do not add up to an obligation to protect any other persons except the patient population with whom this person deals as a health professional. In Case IV, the adverse effects on the teachers, as well as the low utility of the test, advise against this proposed policy.

### 4.2.4 Legal Implications

Most jurisdictions have statutes requiring the physician to report cases of certain sorts, such as sexually transmitted diseases, gunshot and knife wounds and suspected child, partner and elder abuse. These statutes should be obeyed when the physician believes the legal criteria for making a report are met. Some physicians fail to report abuse or venereal disease, particularly when the parents or patients are "respectable." This failure is reprehensible.

In recent years, many jurisdictions have legislated about the confidentiality of HIV testing. The legislation is intended to protect HIV-positive persons from the extreme prejudice that often is directed at them when their condition is known. Usually this legislation does not permit the testing of persons without their explicit consent and requires their consent to share the results with any other party. Exceptions usually allow other health professionals caring for the patient access to the results and permit health officers access to the information for the protection of others. A few states have passed laws that give physicians the discretion whether or not to notify sexual partners of HIV-positive persons. Physicians should be aware of the exact provisions of this legislation in their area.

### 4.3 THE ECONOMICS OF CARE

Costs are incurred whenever medical care is provided. Those costs are paid by patients, by their families, by third-party insurers (public or private) or are subsidized by institutions or individuals. Patients and physicians have always taken costs into account in reaching medical care decisions. It was long assumed that patients would pay the costs of their care and that those who could not pay would be subsidized by the state or the charity of physicians or institutions. The introduction of private and public forms of health insurance changed the economics of health care. More recently, social and political concern to restrain the growth of health costs has had significant impact on the financing of care. Regulatory efforts, such as capitated prospective reimbursement, and market forces, such as proprietary hospital corporations and managed care organizations (MCOs), are seen as mechanisms for constraining costs. The ethical question is how the financing of care, and in particular the cost-containment methods used by these new mechanisms, should influence individual medical decisions. How should the legitimate interests of third parties—health care institutions, insurance companies, labor unions, corporations, government— be factored in to clinical decisions about appropriate care?

Some physicians will say that these interests should not be factored in: their only allegiance is to individual patients; societal or institutional costs are not relevant to clinical decisions. Whatever medical indications and personal preferences require should be provided. An alternative viewpoint is that physicians have both individual and collective responsibility to use limited resources so that fair and efficient care can be provided to all who need it. In this view, clinical judgments should also be microallocation decisions, ideally based on outcome data about cost-effectiveness and on the marginal benefits of an intervention. This view implies that certain patients, despite their preferences may not get every potentially beneficial diagnostic or therapeutic intervention. The physician's dual obligations of allegiance to one's patients and to the welfare of the community must be interpreted in view of contextual factors such as the source of payment, the availability of resources, the seriousness of need, the expectations of insured persons, the solvency of institutions, etc.

### 4.3.1 Costs to Individuals

Some individuals are not covered by public or private health insurance. Many such persons have restricted access to care and probably have poor outcomes in certain chronic diseases. Other persons are able to pay for their own care; in the market system that prevails in American health care, such persons have the opportunities to purchase such care as they desire or the type of health insurance coverage that provides for their needs. This does create some inequity in the allocation of care, since it may siphon dollars and professional talent into forms of medical and surgical care that are luxuries rather than necessities. Still, this is an inequity that our culture tolerates, and even insists upon, in the name of freedom of choice.

### 4.3.2 Emergency Care and Critical Care

Persons who require immediate care for a life-threatening condition may present themselves to a physician or to the emergency department of a hospital. It may be obvious that such persons are uninsured and are unable to pay for the care they need. It is an ancient tenet of medical ethics that physicians should provide services in such situations. The Hippocratic writings state, "If there is an opportunity to serve a stranger in financial straits, give full assistance ... love of humankind and love of the medical art go together." (Precepts VI.) Most emergency care takes place in hospitals. These institutions operate under various legal requirements that mandate emergency care in certain situations. For example, emergency departments are not permitted by law to transfer patients who are medically unstable, and this includes pregnant women in labor. However, in the present economic climate, some hospitals attempt to reduce the financial burden of uncompensated care. Policies developed for this purpose may affect the decisions of physicians working in the institution.

**Case I.** A 28-year-old man was brought to the ER of a rural hospital after an automobile accident in which he suffered head trauma. He was unconscious and his wife, who was not severely injured, informed the admitting nurse that they had no insurance. Evaluation revealed a transtentorial herniation and an acute subdural hematoma. The patient was treated with dexamethasone, mannitol, and phenytoin. Because the rural hospital was not capable of providing neurosurgery, an attempt was made to transfer the patient to University Hospital. When it became clear to University Hospital that the patient lacked medical insurance, the transfer was delayed and the patient died en route to a more distant tertiary care facility.

**Case II.** Metropolitan Hospital is located in an urban area where crime and drug use are rampant. Its neurosurgery service is always busy. A large percentage of its patients are uninsured since, in that state, Medicaid eligibility criteria are high. Other sources of funds for indigent patients are stretched thin. Still, Metropolitan defines its primary mission as service to its local population, including those who are medically indigent. While it accepts emergency patients from outlying areas, it requires proof from distant transfers of ability to pay.

*RECOMMENDATION:*   Physicians who work in institutions that receive emergency patients have an ethical obligation to assure that the traditional medical ethic of service to those in urgent need of care can be fulfilled in their institution. The medical staff must influence hospital policies to this effect. Transfer policies and decisions made in the emergency room must be based on medical indications rather than on financial implications of service in the particular case. It is legitimate for institutions to establish policies that limit the indigent care they provide, but these policies themselves should be consistent with principles of justice. In Case I, the patient's medical indications, requiring immediate neurosurgical intervention, should have been met with a prompt response from University Hospital. The solvency of the institution was not at stake. In Case II, the institution attempted to establish a just policy based on a definition of mission in relationship to its prospects for financial solvency.

**Case III.**   Mr. R.W., a 61-year-old construction worker who has health insurance through his union was transferred from a rural hospital to a tertiary care urban hospital, with a diagnosis of ARDS secondary to *Klebsiella* pneumonia. On presentation, he was comatose and in shock. After four weeks in intensive care, during which he developed many complications, including empyema and a cardiac arrest, he was weaned from the respirator. He was transferred from the ICU to the floor. He recovered without permanent end-organ damage and with good cognitive function. At discharge, his bill was $268,260. On three occasions during his stay in the ICU, the insurance company's case manager asked the attending physician whether there was outcome data to justify continuing the expensive tertiary care.

*COMMENT:*   When tensions arise between providing lifesaving care, based on medical indications and patient preferences (expressed or presumed), and cost-effective care, based on economic considerations, a serious review of medical goals is indicated. If that review confirms the probable utility of treatment, it should be continued. Physicians and payers must realize that any health insurance system involves pooling risk and is designed to balance between cases that lose money and those on whom the insurance company makes money. It is worth noting that the case manager was questioning whether the patient was likely to benefit from the costly interventions. In situations of very high cost, such as this one, the question was reasonable and should encourage physicians to rethink whether their expenditures of money and time can be justified by the goals they are pursuing.

### 4.3.3 Managed Care

In the past decade, new financial arrangements have appeared in medical practice designed to control rising health care costs. Among these are various forms of "managed care" (MC) that is, organizations that integrate the financing and delivery of health care by contracting with health care professionals and hospitals to provide all necessary care to an enrolled population for a fixed annual or monthly premium. This arrangement describes health maintenance organizations (HMOs), but other forms of MC include preferred provider organizations (PPOs) and point-of-service (POS), perhaps the most rapidly increasing segment of the MC market. The percent of people with employer-sponsored health coverage who are enrolled in MC plans rose from 29 percent in 1988 to 73 percent in 1995. The percent of physicians who had signed contracts with MC organizations increased from 61 percent in 1988 to 75 percent in 1993.

HMOs are the most common MC arrangement. Many of these HMOs are for-profit commercial enterprises. The overall income paid by subscribers to the plan is used to pay the expenses of care, administrative costs, and dividends for shareholders. Usually, the physician providers share financial risk for caring for patients. In some plans, physician compensation may vary based on the physician's use of health resources in caring for a panel of patients. Thus, there is an incentive for physicians to be cost-conscious, to stress prevention and even, at times, to balance the patient's needs against the physician's financial incentives. Managed care organizations establish cost-containment measures, such as selection of the population of potential members, the setting of rates and kinds of service, and achieving economies of scale in facilities. Some cost-containment measures directly affect the clinical decisions of physicians working in these settings: physicians are encouraged to make clinical decisions about particular patients that are, on the whole, cost-effective as well as medically appropriate. This may take the unobjectionable form of merely advising physicians to be "cost-conscious," or the more problematic form of providing incentives, such as bonuses or increased portions of the savings accrued, for physicians who reduce costs. Primary among the cost-containment measures is "gatekeeping," namely, the practice of assigning patients to a primary care physician who "manages" their care by selecting the medically appropriate and cost-effective use of procedures, specialty referrals, and hospitalizations. When the role of gatekeeper is combined with financial incentives for underutilizing health resources, the physician is in a potential conflict of interest situation. [Special Issue, Managed Care Ethics. *Arch Intern Med* 1996; 156.]

### 4.3.4 Ethically Acceptable Contracts for Physicians

As managed care becomes the primary organizational structure for delivering health care in the United States, it is important to offer physicians considering working within a managed care system guidelines for an ethically acceptable contractual arrangement. Physicians have an ethical obligation to scrutinize contracts and MCO descriptions for the following:

(a) Quality of Care. In joining an MC plan, physicians must be confident that the organization has the resources, commitment, and ability to provide reasonable health care to its members. A specific definition of "reasonable" will vary based on local needs, practice, and resources. Physicians should ascertain whether the plan's constraints on the availability of procedures reflects sound methods of technology assessment and criteria for quality of care.

(b) Physician Advocacy. Physicians must determine that they can serve without fear of retaliation as advocates for their patients within the constraints of the MC plan. The physician's loyalty to the patient should not extend to advocating for practices that are imprudent, ineffective, or medically inappropriate, but appropriate advocacy must be protected and encouraged.

(c) Patient Choice. Although many employees are not given a choice of health plans, but are required to participate in an MC plan, important aspects of choice should be preserved within the MC program. These include the right of patients to select their primary care physician (who should serve as their advocate rather than as "gatekeeper"); the right to select a specialist such as an obstetrician or cardiologist; and, most important, the right, based on the legal and ethical doctrine of informed consent, to make their own health care decisions.

(d) Full Disclosure. In order for patients to be allowed to make reasonable choices, they must be provided with adequate and truthful information. In the MC setting, this includes information about their illness and the various options for treating it, even if some of these options are not available through the patient's MC plan. It also includes disclosure about the physician's financial incentives that could influence the recommendations the physician makes to the patient. Finally, disclosure must specify those services not covered by the plan, including a clear definition of what is meant by "experimental treatment." Patients should be told they have the right to seek additional care outside of the plan if they are prepared to pay for it "out-of-pocket."

(e) Internal and External Appeals and Grievance Procedures. These mechanisms should be available for both subscribers and physicians within the MCO.

### 4.3.5   Cost Considerations in Reaching Clinical Decisions

In general: (a) patient-centered care that focuses on medical indications and patient preferences should retain priority. This statement merely affirms the traditional responsibility of the physician to place the patient's interest before self-interest and to respect the patient's right of choice. Quality of care should not be subordinated to cost considerations but should be based on clinical data, outcome studies, and practice guidelines. Quality care, however, does not mean all available care. The clinical zeal that does everything for everybody is poor medicine. Medicine that emphasizes the methods of primary care and sound clinical judgment is often the best and most parsimonious medicine. Quality care refers not only to care that is diagnostically sound and technically correct. It must also be rational, that is, no more and no less than reasonably suited to the clinical problem; cost-effective, that is, known to be the least costly way to achieve an equal outcome; and ethical, that is, in accord with ethical criteria, such as those discussed in this book.

(b) The important elements of the patient-physician relationship should be preserved. Managed care has the potential for creating conflicts of interest that divide the physician's allegiance between the patient and the health system, and that place great stress on the patient-physician relationship. The physician's knowledge of the patient and the patient's trust and confidence in the physician must be preserved. This can be achieved by reinforcing the role of the physician as advocate for the patient. MCOs should expect physicians to argue for policies that provide all services that have a reasonable likelihood of benefiting the patient. If the system cannot provide the services, due to limitation of resources, the best case has been made on the patient's behalf. Physicians then have a responsibility to inform patients of these limitations and of the possibility of going outside the plan, at their own cost.

(c) Patient and physician autonomy and freedom of choice should be maximized within the limits of the system. While acknowledging constraints on patient and physician preferences, ways should be devised to maximize autonomy within increasingly complex bureaucratic systems. Persons should be fully informed of the constraints of the system before choosing it. For example, if the plan does not cover "experimental treatment," patients should be given a clear definition of what is meant by "experimental treatment." Also, MC plans should disclose any financial incentive arrangements that exist between the plan and its physicians. To the extent possible, such incentive arrangements should be based on quality of care rather than on underutilization of care services. Physicians should be aware of the plan's quality of care, philosophy of care, and incentive structure before joining it. There should be a formal appeals process where patients' and physicians' views and grievances can be expressed and adjudicated.

(d) The system adopted by any plan should reflect principles of just distribution, such as those mentioned below in 4.4. All participants in a plan, subscribers and providers, should understand and appreciate these principles. Indeed, plans would be wise to invite its members to participate in formulating a philosophy of just care. [Morreim H. *Balancing Act: The New Medical Ethics of Medicine's New Economics*. Boston: Kluwer, 1991; Council of Ethical and Judicial Affairs, American Medical Association. Ethical issues in managed care. *JAMA* 1995; 273:330–335.]

**Case I.**   Mr. S.T., a 52-year-old man with a three-year history of diabetes and a strong family history of ischemic heart disease, complains to his primary physician at an HMO of three weeks of substernal pressure that sometimes occurs at rest. The resting electrocardiogram is normal. The patient requests a referral to a cardiologist, but the primary physician instead orders a multistage exercise test (MSET) but does not include the more sensitive and expensive thallium scintigram for evaluation of chest pain. After a borderline MSET, the patient again insists on a cardiology referral and finally the referral is made. After completing a thallium stress test, which is borderline, the cardiologist decides to treat the patient medically rather than refer the patient to an interventional cardiologist for a coronary angiogram and possible interventions including angioplasty or bypass graft surgery. The HMO to which patient, primary physician, and cardiologist belong is one that distributes a share of the annual profits to physicians if medical care expenditures are kept below a certain level.

*COMMENT:* The primary care physician and cardiologist face conflicts of interest. Their personal financial benefits are based partly on restricting costly services such as thallium scans, coronary angiography, and coronary bypass graft surgery. On the other hand, their professional responsibilities to the patient require that they provide the patient with the best medical or surgical recommendations, even if these involve a costly surgical procedure. If the patient had three-vessel disease, the cardiologist would act unethically and incompetently if she did not recommend surgery. Two-vessel coronary disease and the use of thallium scans are, in contrast, both gray areas in which considerable technical disagreement remains about appropriate use, and wide variation in practice exists. In such circumstances, either decision by the HMO cardiologist would be defensible, but one wonders whether the financial conflict of interest would not incline both the primary care doctor and the cardiologist toward the less expensive alternatives.

*RECOMMENDATION:* Ultimately many of these dilemmas will be resolved by better outcome data. For the present, we must recognize that in gray areas, where physician practice varies, HMO physicians are likely to opt for the least costly alternative. This is ethically defensible, since persons join HMOs for the sake of the financial advantages of membership, as well as in expectation of good care. The financial solvency of such plans is a matter of common interest to all members and hence cost-effective care is in the interests of all. Plan members, however, should be informed that the plan encourages cost-effective care within the context of appropriate care. They should also be told that they can go outside the plan, at their own cost, to seek forms of care that are not recommended or provided within the plan. Public opinion is reacting against some of the more egregious practices of MCOs, such as the "gag rule" and overly restrictive referrals and hospital stays. Medicare and Medicaid regulations and states laws are prohibiting certain other practices, such as direct payment incentives for limiting care. Still, even as MCO practices and policies are made more conformable with the demands of ethics and quality, certain ethical problems will remain.

**Case II.** Mrs. Comfort, the patient with breast cancer, has been a member of a large HMO for seven years. She was first treated for breast cancer three years ago. At that time, she underwent a modified radical mastectomy with reconstruction and an axilliary lymph node dissection that revealed 12 of 19 lymph nodes positive for metastatic disease. Estrogen receptor status was positive. She was subsequently treated with an 8-month course of chemotherapy followed by radiation therapy to the chest wall and has been taking tamoxifen on a daily basis since completion of the radiation and chemotherapy. Mrs. Comfort did well for three years when she noted pain in her thigh. Bone scan revealed multiple metastatic lesions of the long bones and vertebral column. Mrs. Comfort remembered from initial discussions with her oncologist that if her breast cancer recurred, it would probably be incurable. Her oncologist now offered her a choice of either standard palliative chemotherapy, which he said could relieve the pain, or radiation therapy to the sites of bone pain. She elected to receive radiation therapy to the painful bone lesions.

On her own initiative, Mrs. Comfort sought a second opinion from a medical oncologist at a nearby academic medical center. In addition to the two standard treatment options offered by the HMO oncologists, the academic oncologist discussed one other option: high-dose chemotherapy followed by bone marrow transplantation (HDC/BMT).

During the past decade, it was suggested that advanced breast cancer might be cured by administration of extremely high doses of chemotherapy. The dosage was highly toxic and would be fatal without subsequent bone marrow transplantation. Although remission was not uncommon, no data demonstrated a cure rate any greater than conventional chemotherapy. Mrs. Comfort returned to her HMO oncologist and indicated her wish to receive a bone marrow transplantation. Her HMO oncologist discussed this with her and indicated that HDC/BMT was an experimental procedure. He told her that there was considerable discussion in the medical literature about this new intervention and that, on the whole, it appeared that, for persons at her stage of disease, this risky procedure brought occasional remission of disease but showed no evidence of prolonging life. He warned her that there would be difficulties getting the HMO to agree to pay for a transplantation at the local academic medical center. Mrs. Comfort forced the issue by returning to the academic medical center and stating that she wished to participate in the HDC/BMT program. The academic medical center contacted her HMO regarding coverage for the treatment. Initially, the HMO refused to provide coverage. Mrs. Comfort was convinced that HDC/BMT was her last hope. She contacted a lawyer who threatened a suit to force the HMO to provide coverage for the BMT. The HMO, fearing public relations problems and confronted with the prospect of a long and costly court battle, agreed to pay for the cost of the BMT at the academic medical center.

*RECOMMENDATION:* Many centers are now using HDC/BMT as a procedure that may improve patients' quality of life, although there is, as yet, slight data that this procedure prolongs life. In some centers, the procedure is being done as part of a formal clinical research trial, while in other settings, which have extensive experience with it, it is being used as standard treatment. The HMO prefers to regard the procedure as still experimental, which in a sense it is, while the academic oncologist views it as standard care, which in some settings it is. The HMO has a right to exclude experimental procedures from its benefits; if it does so, it must explain clearly to subscribers what that term means and what its consequences for the patient might be. Individual physicians should inform patients of all medical options, including the experimental ones, and give them accurate information about the risks and benefits of each. It appears that this was done eventually in Mrs. Comfort's case. The HMO, however, was in a locale where a research center had extensive experience with HDC/BMT, and results there showed a remission rate higher than in most centers, although no improvement in mortality. The HMO would be wise to enter an agreement with the academic center and offer to its patients the opportunity to volunteer for a randomized trial between HDC/BMT and standard treatment.

**4.4**    ## ALLOCATION OF SCARCE RESOURCES

Allocation of scarce resources is sometimes called "rationing." Rationing can have the broad meaning of distributing any limited resource by any allocation mechanism, such as the market. It may have the more specific meaning of allocating some limited resource by a plan stating criteria and priorities. Gasoline and food rationing in wartime is rationing of this more specific type. Health care in the United States has long been rationed by the market, and in accord with implicit rather than explicit criteria. The number of physicians, the location of their practices, the ability of persons to pay, the different perceptions of medical need— these factors and many others result in medical resources being allocated in certain ways. Various sorts of financial and administrative arrangements can result in certain allocations and constitute implicit rationing. In recent years, the question has been raised whether medical resources should be allocated by explicit criteria: the state of Oregon established priorities according to which particular treatments for particular disease conditions would be reimbursed by Medicaid. This question belongs to the ethics of health policy and is not discussed in this book. However, any such policy will have effects at the clinical level. The question will quickly arise whether physicians should make allocation decisions by balancing societal efficiency against the interests of individual patients. [EB: "Health Care Resources, Allocation of," II, 1067–1183: PBE: "Allocation, Rationing," ch. 6, 361–386; ME: Buchanan A. "Health Care Delivery and Resource Allocation," ch. 11, 321–362; Kilner JF. *Who Lives? Who Dies? Ethical Criteria in Patient Selection*. New Haven: Yale University Press, 1990.]

**Case.**    Mr. D.P., a 69-year-old man with a long history of heart disease and diabetes is admitted to an ICU with fever, hypotension, and shortness of breath. The chest film is consistent with ARDS, and the $P_{O_2}$ is 50. At morning rounds, the intern asks whether this aggressive, costly treatment is appropriate for an elderly man who has underlying heart disease and diabetes and whose chances of recovering unimpaired from this episode may be no greater than 35 percent. At the noon staff conference, the attending physician distributes an essay written by a prominent public official that states:

> We've got a duty to die and get out of the way with all our machines and artificial hearts and everything like that, and let our other society, our kids, build a reasonable life. No one who is otherwise healthy should die of a curable disease. On the other hand, no one with a terminal disease should receive endless treatment if the marginal benefits far exceed the costs. The economic reality is that every dollar spent on health care is a dollar we can't spend to retool America, improve our schools or replace our infrastructure. Medical science can make individuals well, but it also can make our nation economically sick. We are forced to make choices. Do we provide all the extraordinary medical care desperately ill people can take or do we improve our school systems, repair our roads, bridges, dams, and other public facilities?

The attending asks the house officers whether these ideas apply to Mr. D.P. Should they provide indicated treatment or should they begin rationing health care by making tough choices, starting immediately with this 69-year-old man?

*COMMENT:* The easiest form of rationing for individual physicians—and the least problematic ethically—involves forgoing medical activities that are useless or unnecessary. Costly, scarce resources should not be expended wastefully on patients who will not benefit. This is an ethical obligation of physicians. Of course, determining when a particular form of intervention is likely to be useless, unnecessary or only marginally beneficial requires acute clinical judgment and is often impossible. The recent trend toward outcome studies and clinical epidemiology can be helpful. However, the clinician must base clinical judgments on medical indications and patient preferences, and less on quality-of-life factors such as age, mental status, or financial resources. The public official quoted is correct when he states: "No one with a terminal disease should receive endless treatment if the marginal benefits far exceed the costs." The problem, as illustrated in the case of the 69-year-old man (who subsequently recovered without any impairment), is that at the time of his admission to the hospital, physicians could not be certain whether they were dealing with someone who was "terminally ill" or whether they were dealing with someone, as the case turned out, who was critically ill but had great hopes of recovering completely.

### 4.4.1 Admission to Programs with Limited Resources

Medical care is so organized that certain procedures and therapeutic programs are available only at a few locales or from a few specialists. More persons may need this sort of care than can be accommodated. How should the resources be allocated? All commentators on the ethics of this problem agree that resources should be allocated in a fair manner. What constitutes fairness?

*EXAMPLE:*   When chronic hemodialysis became available in the 1960s, the very limited resources required some rationing device. A local committee was established to screen all applicants who had been judged acceptable on medical grounds. The committee relied on "social worth" criteria, that is, personal and social characteristics that merited the treatment. This technique proved unworkable and was much criticized for bias and prejudice.

*COMMENT:*   Extensive ethical discussion of this issue seems to have reached consensus on the unacceptability of social worth as a principle of fair distribution. Some commentators have favored "queuing" (first come, first served), although they note that these systems favor the better informed and better connected, who can hurry to the queue. Many favor a lottery, whereby all participate in a drawing of random numbers. This system, however, is faulted because all the pool of needy persons does not exist at any one time. In the most extensive program requiring allocation of scarce resources, organ transplantation, selection is now facilitated by the international computerized system for tissue typing. This introduces a major objective consideration, which obviates the biases of social worth and also reduces the uneasiness of having life and death depend purely on "the luck of the draw."

The dangers of bias and prejudice inherent in a social worth system advise its rejection as a rationing device. It seems most fair to establish certain basic objective criteria—for example, medical condition, potential for benefit, and age—and within a pool of those who meet these criteria to select randomly. It may also be useful to establish a "due process" system, which could make exceptions to these criteria. Exceptions should be based on the "triage" principles.

Access to organ transplantation for those who medically qualify for it is problematic. First, due to a shortage of usable organs for transplantation, the demand far exceeds the supply. For example, in the United States only about 16,000 solid-organ—kidney, heart, liver, lung—transplants are performed each year. Yet approximately 25,000 people are on a national waiting list. Second, even if a person is medically eligible for a transplant, he or she may lack the money necessary to purchase it. For example, heart and liver transplants require as much as $150,000 for the initial surgery. Persons whose insurance does not cover it or who lack personal wealth do not get a transplant. Third, some persons who may medically need an organ transplant may be ineligible on other grounds, such as being an incarcerated criminal for whom such services are not made available. Lack of access to medically indicated treatment extends to many other populations, including schizophrenics, AIDS patients, or others who cannot afford expensive medications. Access to care for persons with no or inadequate health insurance is limited to what they can obtain through emergency care. Persons who suffer from catastrophic injury or illness often lack resources for long-term hospitalization or rehabilitation. Allocation of and access to health care resources are continuing problems of social justice. [ME: "Organ Transplantation," ch. 9, 239–274; EB: "Organ and Tissue Procurement" and "Organ and Tissue Transplants," IV, 1852–1874.]

### 4.4.2 Triage

Medical care has long been provided in accord with a rationing plan in one specific situation, battlefield medicine. In recent years triage rules have been refined and applied to other disasters, such as earthquakes and hurricanes. The rules of triage and its rationale are stated in a handbook of military surgery:

> Priority is to be given to (1) slightly injured who can be quickly returned to service, (2) the more seriously injured who demand immediate resuscitation or surgery, (3) the "hopelessly wounded" or the dead on arrival ... The military surgeon must expend his energies in the treatment of only those whose survival seems likely, in line with the objective of military medicine, which has been defined as "doing the greatest good for the greatest number" in the proper time and place. [*Emergency War Surgery*. Washington, D.C.: Government

Printing Office, 1958; EB: "Triage," V, 2496–2498; Winslow GR. *Triage and Justice.* Berkeley: University of California Press, 1982.]

*COMMENT:*    The ethical basis for military triage is to return to service those who are needed for victory, a common good for the army and the nation. Similarly, disaster triage provides priority to persons such as firefighters, public safety officers, and medical personnel in order for them to be returned to rescue work. Present disaster and serious danger to the society justify triage rules. Lacking the element of present disaster and the destruction of the fabric of social order, rules that subordinate the needs of individuals to the needs of society are not easily justified in medical ethics. However, recent debates over allocation of organs for transplantation have invoked a version of the triage principle.

More than 7,000 people in the United States are currently on the liver transplantation waiting list and 10 people die each day because a donor organ is not available. In the face of such dire scarcity, the United Network on Organ Sharing (UNOS) announced a major change in policy whereby livers would now be allocated first to critically ill patients with acute liver failure rather than to comparably ill persons with chronic liver disease who had been waiting on the list for a longer time. The rationale for deciding to place acute liver failure patients ahead of those with chronic disease—essentially allowing them to "jump the queue"—was based on the triage concept that in a situation of dire scarcity the sickest persons with the highest survival chances were to be transplanted first. Thus, priority would be given to patients with acute liver disease who generally had fewer comorbid conditions and thus a higher likelihood of survival than patients with chronic disease. [EB: "Organ and Tissue Procurement," IV, 1852–1871; ME: "Organ Transplantation," ch. 9, 239–274.]

### 4.4.3    Competing Claims to Care
Situations arise when it can be asked whether the claims of one patient for care override the claims of another. Personnel, time, equipment, beds, and other factors are insufficient to accommodate both. In addition, fundamental ethical justification for triage, namely, contribution to social good, is not present; this is a competition between two rival claimants.

**Case 1.** Mrs. C.Z. is a 71-year-old woman who has a diagnosed lung tumor for which she refused surgery. She developed obstructive pneumonia and was admitted to the community hospital in her rural county. She has shown no signs of improvement for seven days. She is comatose. The victim of an automobile accident is brought to the hospital with a crushed chest, apparent pneumothorax, and broken bones in the extremities. The patient requires a respirator immediately. Mrs. C.Z., of the six patients on the six respirators in the unit, has the poorest prognosis. She seems unable to be weaned and thus would probably die if ventilatory support was discontinued. Should she be removed in favor of the accident victim?

*COMMENT:* The medical prognosis of Mrs. C.Z. is poor. She has cancer of the lung with broncheal obstruction and pneumonia that has failed to respond to treatment. She is comatose and likely to die within days. Nothing is known about her preferences, except her refusal of surgery. Given these considerations, the immediate and serious need of an identifiable other person becomes an important consideration. When that person is in imminent danger of death, the contextual factor of scarcity of resources becomes decisive in the decision regarding Mrs. C.Z. It is ethically permissible to recommend that respiratory support be discontinued.

**Case II.** Patient R.A., the drug addict described in 2.9.2, is in need of a second prosthetic heart valve. Several physicians are strongly opposed to providing a second prosthesis. These physicians offer three reasons: (1) surgery is futile, since the patient will become reinfected; (2) the patient does not care enough about himself to follow a regimen or to abstain from drugs; (3) it is a poor use of societal resources.

*COMMENT:* The first and second considerations are discussed in 1.2.2 and in 2.9.2. The third consideration raises new ethical issues. (a) What are the criteria for differentiating good from poor uses of societal resources? While such criteria might be formulated at the policy level, it is impossible to do so at the clinical level: the overall view of social need and the contribution of particular decisions to that need are not known to clinicians. Also, as we noted in 3.0.8, attempts to formulate such criteria run the danger of introducing serious bias and discrimination into clinical decisions.

(b) There is no guarantee that whatever is "saved" by refusing this patient will be used in any better manner.

(c) The resources are, of course, not being "absorbed" by the patient; they are flowing to the hospital, to the physicians and surgeons, to nurses and so on. Blame for "wasting" resources may be better laid on the system than the patient.

*RECOMMENDATION:* The most acceptable ethical justification for refusing to provide a second prosthesis is the medical indication that the risks of surgery and its attendant mortality exceed the risks of managing the patient with medical therapy. Thus, if medically indicated, the surgery should be offered. The ethical obligation to provide surgical assistance is, however, diminished to the extent that the rights of other patients are directly compromised, as explained in Comment to Case I.

### 4.4.4 P  Organ Transplantation for Children

Successful organ transplantation depends on having donors that are HLA compatible. Such donors are often siblings. Thus, questions may occasionally arise about taking a kidney or bone marrow from a healthy child for a seriously ill sibling. This question had an inauspicious answer when first asked, since the healthy child was retarded, thus raising the suspicion that the retarded are to be disvalued and used for the benefit of others. However, the major question is the risk to which a healthy child is put for the possible benefit of another. In our view, it is indefensible to impose the serious risk of removal of a kidney; it is defensible to suggest the notably less serious risks of donation of bone marrow. Needless to say, the negotiations with family and with the child require the utmost delicacy, the psychological implications for the children in the event of either failure or success, must be recognized, and the legal requirements in the jurisdiction must be complied with. Should there be parental disagreement, the plan should be abandoned.

**Case I.**   An anencephalic infant is born. The parents request that the infant be resuscitated and ventilated long enough to remove organs for transplantation.

*COMMENT:*   The harvesting of organs from anencephalic infants is ethically questionable, since they are not, at the time of removal of organs, dead by brain criteria (1.5.1 P). This violates the important moral principle of not using one human as a means to the welfare of another without consent. Even though legislation might approve the removal of organs from living anencephalics, the prospect of extending this practice to other unwilling, dying subjects should give pause. The proposal has not been favored in the ethical literature. [Peabody JL, Jonsen AR. Organ Transplantation. In: Goldworth A, Silverman W, Stevenson DK, Young EWD. *Ethics and Perinatology.* New York: Oxford University Press, 1994.]

**Case II.**   A woman is pregnant with a fetus diagnosed in the early second trimester as having anomalies incompatible with life. She is asked by a researcher whether tissue from her aborted fetus can be used for a research project, the implantation of fetal pancreatic tissue in adult diabetic patients.

*COMMENT:*   The transplantation of fetal tissue for the reversal of diabetes and Parkinson's disease is presently a research procedure. It is not research on the fetus, since the research subject is the adult patient. The tissue may be used (a) if no direct connection exists between the abortion and the obtaining of the tissue, (b) maternal consent is obtained, (c) a research protocol has been approved by the local IRB.

**4.5**                              **THE LAW**

The law has been mentioned many times in this book on ethics. The practice of medicine has long been the subject of legislation, and many judicial cases have involved medical practice, particularly when physicians are accused of negligence. In recent years, the volume of legislation, litigation, and regulation around medicine and health care has increased notably. In certain areas, such as the care of the terminally ill patient, legal and ethical issues are closely related. Judicial decisions, such as those listed in 3.3.1, have been handed down. The Supreme Court of the United States has alluded to a constitutionally protected "liberty interest" that supports a person's right to refuse medical care, even when life-sustaining (3.3.1) and spoken on the constitutionality of assisted suicide

(3.5.5). Administrative regulations, such as the Regulations for Protection of Human Subjects of Research or the Baby Doe Rules, are in force. The question is what place these various sorts of law have in ethical decision-making and, more acutely, what to do when a legal rule seems to contradict an ethical imperative.

Statutes passed by legislatures, such as Natural Death Acts, the Uniform Definition of Death Act, and the Uniform Anatomical Gift Act, enable medical decisions to be made without fear of liability. They facilitate legally certain decisions and practices that have been judged ethically acceptable, yet might be judged legally perilous without special provision of the law (2.6). Some laws and regulations impose limits on decisions that appear ethically appropriate to those involved in the case.

*EXAMPLES:* (a) Discontinuing nutrition and hydration for a patient in a persistent vegetative state is now widely accepted as ethical (3.2.3), yet some states have specific legislation that prohibits doing so and others have legislation that requires "clear and convincing evidence" that the patient would have chosen this course.

(b) A jurisdiction might enact laws or regulations that require extensive procedural steps before a DNAR order can be written. Cases may occur in which DNAR might seem medically appropriate, yet all procedural steps have not been completed.

(c) A jurisdiction might enact laws and regulations that limit access to certain medical resources for certain classes of persons. For example, Medicaid recipients might not be eligible for major organ transplants.

*COMMENT:* The legal context of medical decisions must be evaluated in terms of the nature of the law and the nature of the case. In (a), legal challenge to the law is a recourse open to families, physicians and institutions. In (b), a physician may choose to act contrary to the law, in the name of professional ethics, carefully document the rationale for the decision, and take the risk of exposure to legal liability. The problem posed in (c) is discussed at 4.0.2 and 4.4.

In general, codes of professional ethics define appropriate conduct as being within the confines of the law. For example, with regard to confidentiality, all information obtained in the course of providing medical care is deemed confidential except disclosures required or permitted by law. Physicians may sometimes feel frustrated by laws that seem burdensome, such as reporting requirements or limitations on access to care. In specific cases physicians may, seek authorization for making an exception to usual legal requirements or seek clarification of their precise legal obligations. Sometimes physicians falsely believe or assert that the law imposes duties that are not required. Also, some physicians have an inordinate and uninformed fear of liability. Studies have shown that physicians generally receive their legal knowledge from highly unreliable sources, namely, from other physicians. When questions arise about legal regulation of medical practice, it is prudent to seek expert advice. When questions arise about potential conflicts between ethical values and legal obligations, physicians should utilize institutional means—such as ethics consultation, or committees, legal services, professional organizations—to clarify their options and responsibilities. [McCracy SV, Swanson JW, Perkins HS, Winslade WJ. Treatment decisions for terminally ill patients: physicians' legal defensiveness and knowledge of medical law. *Law, Medicine & Health Care* 1992; 20:364–376.]

### 4.5.1 P  Law and Pediatrics

Certain laws particularly affect the care of infants and children. All states have passed child protection legislation which requires providers to report to authorities instances of suspected abuse and neglect of children. Two federal laws, one statutory and the other judicial, also pertain to clinical decisions made by pediatricians. In 1985, the U.S. Congress passed amendments to The Child Abuse Prevention and Treatment and Adoption Reform Act. These amendments, commonly known as the "Baby Doe Rules," set certain legal standards for clinical decisions regarding the care of the newborn infant. We have mentioned these rules under the topics where they apply (1.4.2 P, 2.7.8 P, 3.0.10 P). The Baby Doe Rules are not addressed directly to providers of neonatal care: they apply to State Child Protective Agencies, which are required to monitor their observance by hospitals. Neonatologists are advised to seek interpretation of these rules from local legal counsel.

A recent controversial court decision about medical care for an anencephalic infant was based on federal legislation designed to guarantee appropriate emergency care for indigent patients. Baby K was born anencephalic. Her mother, who had strong, religiously based vitalistic beliefs, chose to take her home for the remainder of her expected short life. When the baby experienced, as would be expected, serious respiratory distress, the mother brought her to the hospital emergency department for treatment. Although reluctant to provide treatment that the physicians judged futile, the hospital did so, but then petitioned the court for relief. The court found that the federal Emergency Medical Treatment and Active Labor Act (EMTALA), a federal law requiring hospitals to stabilize emergency patients before transferring them, obliged the hospital to provide medical care for Baby K. In this case, the mother's beliefs and hopes prevailed over the hospital's claim that continued ventilator support was futile. It is difficult to generalize from this peculiar case to the broad problem of defining the futility of treatment (1.2.2).

**4.6**                          **RESEARCH**

Clinical research is essential to modern medicine: new therapeutic and diagnostic interventions must be tested and evaluated by applying them to humans, and often those humans must be patients, persons suffering from the disease for which the intervention is designed. In the past, patients were often unwilling and unknowing subjects of clinical research. Today, this is ethically and legally unacceptable: research is clearly distinguished from treatment. Physicians must know how that distinction is made and be aware of their responsibilities when they undertake clinical research. [EB: "Research, Human," IV, 2248–2256; ME: Capron AM. "Human Experimentation," ch. 6, 135–185; Levine RJ. *Ethics and Regulation of Clinical Research,* New Haven: Yale University Press, 1986.]

**4.6.1    Definition of Clinical Reåsearch**

Clinical research is defined as any clinical intervention involving human subjects, patients or normal volunteers, performed in accord with a protocol designed to yield generalizable scientific knowledge. The protocol sets out the research techniques, such as randomization and double blinding, as well as the statistical techniques necessary to establish validity of the data. The benefits of research accrue to persons other than the subject of research, namely, to future patients, to the professional doing the research, and to society in general. Even when the subject personally benefits—for example, a cancer goes into remission as the result of treatment with an experimental drug—these others benefit from the knowledge produced by the research.

## 4.6.2 Regulation of Clinical Research

Clinical research is governed by guidelines stated in several ethical codes (Nuremberg, Helsinki, American Medical Association). Regulations promulgated by the U.S. Department of Health and Human Services are mandatory for all research carried out in institutions that receive federal funds and also for research done in private industry that will be submitted for FDA approval. [45 Code of Federal Regulations 46:1981; 48:1983.]

These regulations require:

(a) Review of proposed research by an institutional review board (IRB). The IRB is made up of persons competent to understand the science of the protocol, as well as other informed persons, some of whom should be independent of the institution. This IRB must evaluate the design of the protocol, assess the risks and benefits of the research procedures, and recommend approval or disapproval to the funding agency. Many of the ethical problems regarding research must be resolved in the course of the review, for example, an appropriate risk/benefit ratio, the details of informed consent, the suitability of compensation.

(b) Informed consent by any competent participant or permission by guardians for decisionally incapacitated persons (with special review and protection procedures for specific cases). Consent must stress the voluntary nature of participation in research and indicate that the patient's refusal will not compromise the care and attention due to all patients. Coercion, due to excessive compensation or to the professional authority of the researcher, must be avoided.

(c) Fair selection of subjects. Attention must be paid to the selection of appropriate populations as research subjects, that is, researchers must avoid taking advantage of vulnerable populations and must achieve racial and gender balance, to the extent compatible with the objectives of the protocol.

## 4.6.3 Investigational and Innovative Treatment

Most clinical activity involves familiar procedures and medications; relatively few of these have undergone the close scrutiny of a formally designed clinical trial. Their efficacy is attested only by cumulative experience. New treatments are constantly being devised by commercial firms and by individual physicians.

*EXAMPLE:* Physicians may choose to employ a drug, which has FDA approval for one indication, for another condition in which it has never been used ("off label use"). Surgeons may modify a standard surgical maneuver or create an entirely new one.

*COMMENT:* Clinicians may employ such methods in the care of a particular patient. They should do so prudently, with solid assurance that the new use or procedure is likely to be safe and effective. This is called "innovative treatment." It is not research because the use is not designed to produce generalizable information, even though a clinician might be able to draw conclusions in retrospect. Innovative treatment is not, as such, governed by the codes and regulations that govern research. However, it should be governed by the same spirit. The advice of knowledgeable colleagues should be sought, a risk/benefit ratio as accurate as possible should be worked out, and the consent of the patient to be the recipient of yet untried treatment should be obtained. In addition, innovative treatment should be designed as closely as possible to research, so that the social benefit of valid knowledge can be obtained. Finally, in doubtful cases, clinicians should seek the advice of the IRB about the advisability of innovative treatment. Misjudgment in using innovative treatment can lead to malpractice charges.

"Investigational treatment" describes forms of diagnosis and therapy that are under development and have not reached the stage where a formally designed clinical trial can demonstrate efficacy. Development is fostered because existing data suggest that the treatment is "promising." Patients suffering from a condition for which no effective therapy exists may seek such promising treatment, and their physicians, even if skeptical about its efficacy, may be eager to offer hope. Third-party payers usually explicitly exclude investigational (sometimes called "experimental") treatment from coverage and managed care organizations discourage its use.

*EXAMPLE:* We mentioned above, at 4.3.5, the procedure known as high-dose chemotherapy with bone marrow transplantation (HDC/BMT). Many women sought this treatment although it was still investigational. Insurers consistently refused to pay for it, invoking the experimental or investigational exclusion clause of their contracts. A number of successful lawsuits instigated by women seeking the procedure gradually forced HMOs and insurers to pay for it. It became difficult to obtain the needed data about the efficacy of this procedure. This example reveals a conflict between autonomy and justice: individual demands are honored to the detriment of future patients.

*COMMENT:* Investigational treatments should be recommended with great caution. Their promise is often unfulfilled, their negative effects sometimes hidden. At the same time, patients may have no other recourse, and medicine advances by these tentative steps. Physicians should make every effort to assure that their patients see these treatments in a realistic light. Administrators of health plans should make clear the policy of their organization relative to provision and reimbursement and establish means of assessing treatment.

**4.6.4    Ethical Problems in Clinical Research**

All clinician-researchers should honor the ethics of clinical research by abiding by the requirements of informed consent of subjects and review of protocols by competent bodies. However, in clinical situations ethical problems may still arise. It might be asked whether a particular patient, who is in general an appropriate candidate for an approved protocol, should be approached because the risk/benefit ratio is questionable in this patient's case. This problem might arise in situations in which a new drug, believed to be of potential benefit from preliminary animal and human investigations, is compared in a formal clinical trial against a placebo.

Randomized clinical trials are essential to the development of effective and safe medical (and surgical) therapies. In double-blind trials, neither the doctor nor the patient knows whether the patient is receiving a drug or placebo. Some physicians find this situation clinically and ethically unacceptable. Some physicians are concerned that their patients may be randomized to an inferior therapy. However, a properly designed controlled trial would be one in which a true null hypothesis exists so that neither of the proposed therapies could be regarded as definitely better than the other. Also, prejudice about efficacy can cause serious harm. Early neonatology provides a tragic example. When administration of high dosages of oxygen was suspected as the cause of retrolental fibroplasia, a randomized trial was resisted because of the conviction, unconfirmed by evidence, that high dosage was necessary for effective therapy. It can be asked whether patients should be continued on protocol, or new patients entered, when a clinician-researcher believes the majority of patients whom he has treated seem to benefit from one experimental drug rather than the standard treatment.

*EXAMPLE I.* A clinician is entering patients in a randomized double-blind trial of a drug to prevent angina. He suspects from the side effects which drug is the standard one and which the experimental. He also has the impression that patients on the suspected research drug are doing much better.

*COMMENT:* The investigator seems caught between two obligations, the duty to benefit the patient and the contractual duty to carry out the trial (and the more abstract duty to advance medical science). In principle, the duty to benefit the patient supersedes all others. However, in this situation, suspicion and clinical impression do not override the scientifically founded uncertainty when properly collected data are analyzed. Only if the individual clinical investigator is convinced that the use or nonuse of a certain drug may cause harm does it become unethical to proceed. Soundly designed clinical trials should have oversight mechanisms to monitor trends, to deal with the problems of clinical impressions, and to terminate the trial should the evidence of distinct benefit or harm become pervasive.

*EXAMPLE II.* A new drug is being tested to determine its efficacy in treatment of cytomegalovirus (CMV) retinitis, a frequent infection of persons with AIDS and one that can result in blindness. A strictly controlled trial has been designed to gather the most valid data possible, since the known adverse effects of the drug must be balanced by demonstrated benefits. One aspect of the control is a random allocation of patients into two groups, one of which will receive the new drug and the other a combination of the two best of the currently used drugs. A physician involved in the trial finds that certain of her patients specifically request the new drug on the grounds that AIDS advocacy literature indicates that it is more effective in preventing blindness. She wonders whether she should provide the drug outside of the controlled trial.

*COMMENT:* The investigator should not provide the drug outside the trial. The trial is based on the hypothesis that the new drug and the old drugs are equivalent; the outcome of the trial will demonstrate the superiority of one over the other, based on clinical efficacy and drug toxicity. The investigator should disabuse those who seek the experimental drug of the idea that it will give them a better chance. Use of the drug outside the trial will confound the evidence necessary to demonstrate the utility of the new drug.

### 4.6.5 P Pediatric Research

The involvement of children as research subjects was carefully studied by the National Commission for the Protection of Subjects of Biomedical and Behavioral Research. The conclusions of that commission are now embodied in federal regulations that reflect sound ethical judgments. In addition to the ethical considerations about research in general, stated in 4.6, pediatric research should be based on the following ethical principles: [Department of Health and Human Services Rules and Regulations. 45 Code of Federal Regulations 46, subpart D: 1983.]

(a) There must be sound reasons why the research must be done with children. In general, this will be because the condition under study affects only children, and no animal models suffice to study it. The results should be important for the health of children.

(b) The level of risk to the child must be carefully determined. If the risk of research is nonexistent or minimal, that is, not exceeding the risks allowed children in daily life or the risks of routine medical care, there need be no prospect of benefit to the child to justify the research. If the risks are more than minimal, some prospect of personal benefit must be present, that is, the research must also have some therapeutic potential for the subject.

(c) Any research proposal that involves more than minimal risks and offers no personal benefit to the subject requires special review in order to adjudicate its vital importance for the health of children. Institutional review boards, which must approve of all research, can advise researchers about details of the requirements for ethical research involving children.

(d) The informed consent of parents or guardians, and their close involvement in the research, must be obtained. The consent of the child should also be sought when the child is at that stage of maturity where the nature of the procedure and the concept of an invitation to help others voluntarily can be understood. A child's dissent should be respected unless the research procedure is directly associated with a necessary therapy that cannot be provided outside research modalities.

(e) Research on the human fetus should be limited to activities directed to the health of the fetus and should be only of minimal risk. [Tyson J, Beauchamp TL. The boundary between therapeutic and non-therapeutic research; Silverman WA, Goldworth A. Informed consent. In: Goldworth A, et al. *Ethics and Perinatology*. New York: Oxford University Press, 1995.]

**Case.**   Amy, the girl with acute myelogenous leukemia (1.2.4 P), received a bone marrow transplantation, after which she relapsed. Amy is a candidate for a clinical research protocol of a new drug combination. She is now 11 years old. Her parents are eager to enter into the trial. She repeatedly and tearfully refuses.

*COMMENT:*   Therapy and research are significantly different. Therapy promises sound hope of achieving the goal of intervention; research may offer some hope of doing so, but also has as its goal the benefit of other and future patients. A refusal of research by a child, even if it might be thought that the child, if older, would accept, should generally be honored. The National Commission for the Protection of Human Subjects of Biomedical and Behavioral Research recommended that age 7 be considered as the point at which a child's consent for a research intervention be sought and refusal honored. This has been criticized as unrealistic, but it emphasizes the point that children have the right to refuse interventions that hold more promise for others than for themselves.

## 4.7                    TEACHING INVOLVING
##                        PATIENT COOPERATION

Many patients receive care in institutions where clinical teaching is done. Their disease and its diagnosis and treatment provide an opportunity for students in the health sciences to learn the skills necessary for their profession. Often, treatment will be provided by a student. It is possible that some clinical decisions are made with a view to teaching and that such decisions may conflict with the patient's interests and/or wishes.

### 4.7.1    Consent to Be a Teaching Subject
Persons who enter teaching hospitals usually sign a general consent to that effect. Many patients, particularly those who are seriously ill at the time of admission or who for other reasons are

unable to comprehend the meaning of the teaching hospital consent form, have probably not given adequate informed consent to be used as teaching subjects. They should be asked specifically about each episode of teaching and invited to participate. The fact that a particular procedure will be done by a student, and that it is for teaching rather than for their care or in addition to their care, should be made clear. The request should be made politely and a refusal accepted graciously. Patients are amazingly generous in consenting to participate in the education of medical students in teaching hospitals.

On occasion of the history taking and physical diagnosis course, many patients provide their histories to five or more students without complaint. In the light of these observations, it is particularly important that, when the occasional patient refuses to participate in one or another teaching exercise, the student and the faculty respect the patient's wishes absolutely and not threaten or intimidate the patient in any way. Medical students and physicians must remember that individual patients are not obligated to participate in the training of society's future physicians. They almost invariably are eager to do so, and physicians should be sensitive to their enormous debt to patients for patients' unquestioning generosity.

**Case I.**   A 52-year-old obese woman required a lumbar puncture. She had, on admission, signed a general consent to teaching procedures that did not specify who would perform them. A second-year resident entered her room with two medical students. He told the patient that she needed a procedure, positioned her and, when she was turned toward the wall, handed the syringe to the medical student, indicating that she was to draw the spinal fluid. The student had seen the resident perform the procedure on the previous day. The resident then left the room. After several unsuccessful attempts, one medical student sought the resident who, on returning, said "you've got to learn!"

*COMMENT:*   There is no ethical problem in this case; it is an ethical outrage. No consideration was shown to the patient's feelings, appropriate informed consent was not obtained, supervision was inadequate, easily arranged accommodations were not made. Students are often offended by being placed in such situations. As low persons in the medical school hierarchy, students may feel an ethical conflict and not know how, and to whom, to express their feelings.

Although the case described is an ethical outrage rather than an ethical problem, we must be aware that relatively inexperienced students perform many procedures in teaching hospitals, including blood drawing, intravenous insertions, lumbar punctures, paracenteses, thoracenteses, and occasional endotracheal intubations. Students often remark (in private) about their feelings concerning these procedures. They are eager to learn these skills and believe they must master these techniques in order to function effectively as physicians. Still, they are not sure how to approach the patient and how much disclosure is appropriate for the patient's informed consent, particularly for relatively innocuous, albeit discomforting, procedures, such as venipuncture.

Any senior person who orders a student to perform a clinical procedure assumes responsibility for the safe execution of the procedure and for its consequences. Senior persons should invite students to express their discomfort or doubts about what they are asked to do.

**Case II.** A 74-year-old man with chronic obstructive pulmonary disease is admitted in mild respiratory failure with diffuse bronchospasm. His respiratory condition does not require insertion of a Swan-Ganz catheter for hemodynamic monitoring. Nevertheless, the chief resident suggests a catheter be placed; one of her reasons for this choice is to allow an inexperienced intern to practice this technical procedure.

*COMMENT:* Procedures involving any risk should be performed only for diagnostic or therapeutic purposes. Risky procedures should not be done exclusively or even partially for their teaching value. Thus, in Case II, the intern's need for additional practice should not affect the chief resident's clinical judgment. If the procedure is harmless, such as palpation or auscultation, or involves only minor inconvenience, such as asking a patient with ataxic gait to get up from a chair and walk across the room, or minor discomfort, as extension and flexing of an arthritic limb, patients may be requested to allow the procedure. Noninvasive procedures involving neither risk nor discomfort, such as auscultation or examination of pupils or skin, are permitted even on patients who are decisionally incapacitated.

**Case III.**  A second-year medical student is being mentored by a surgeon in private practice. A patient has been prepared for an appendectomy and is now under anesthesia. The surgeon suggests that the student might do his first pelvic examination on the unconscious patient.

*COMMENT:*  This is ethically unacceptable. The patient has not consented to this particularly intimate procedure and, even though unconscious, suffers an offense to her dignity. The student is embarrassed, both at doing the examination and at expressing his discomfort to his mentor. Medical schools should have careful guidelines on this subject and, if possible, arrange teaching experiences that are acceptable to students and to patients.

## 4.7.2  Teaching Procedures on the Newly Dead

Many teaching programs use recently dead patients to teach various nonmutilating procedures including tracheal intubation, placement of central venous catheters, and pericardiocentesis. In one study, only 10 percent of the programs that used newly dead patients for teaching obtained either verbal or written consent from the patient's survivors. Proponents of training on the newly dead argue that it is beneficial to society, nonmutilating to the dead patient, and that there are no good alternatives. They further argue that consent need not be sought because the grieving survivors should not be further troubled about something that is not harmful or mutilating to their deceased relative. It is our opinion that, while the newly dead may be used to teach some procedures, it is ethically and legally appropriate to seek consent from next of kin. Consent acknowledges that we recognize and respect the special status of the newly dead person; omitting consent is a violation of trust. Many families have religious or cultural beliefs that should be respected; and also, secretive activities are offensive to many health professionals, including medical students, nurses, and society. Finally, a number of studies have shown that consent for procedures such as endotracheal intubation can frequently be obtained from family if approached in a sensitive and respectful manner. [McNamara RM, Monti S, Kelley JJ. Requesting consent for an invasive procedure in newly deceased adults. *JAMA* 1995; 273: 310–312; Orlowski JP, Kanoti GA, Mehlman MJ. The ethics of using newly dead patients for teaching and practicing intubation techniques. *NEJM* 1988; 391:439–441.]

**OCCUPATIONAL MEDICINE**

The occupational physician, the military physician, and the prison or police physician may encounter conflicts of interest. As physicians they are obligated to serve those who come to them as patients; as employees they have some obligations to their employers. Ethical problems may arise, particularly about confidentiality and disclosure. [EB: "Occupational Health and Safety," IV, 1838-1851; Rosenstock L, Hagopian A. Ethical dilemmas in providing health care to workers. *Ann Intern Med* 1987; 107: 580.]

**Case I.**   The dialysis nurse described in 4.2.3 is examined by the hospital's Employee Health Service physician. This examination is required by hospital regulations. When the physician tells the nurse she is hepatitis B antigen-positive, she insists he not report her to the director of the dialysis unit.

*COMMENT:*   The physician in this case has accepted responsibilities to the institution as well as responsibilities to particular patients. This dual relationship should be clear to the patient in this situation. The physician should report this patient. The dual relationship may not be clear in many situations where workers approach company physicians. It is imperative that the dual relationship be made clear whenever it is relevant and that its implications be spelled out for a patient-employee.

**Case II.**   A worker in an industry using kepone visits the company physician about a persistent cough. The physician does a cursory physical and prescribes a cough medicine. It is company policy not to investigate symptoms of this sort too aggressively until they become demonstrably more serious. It is also policy not to suggest to worker-patients the potential for lung disease or to make employee health records available to them.

*COMMENT:*   The company policy is manifestly unethical since it causes persons who may be benefited by early diagnosis and treatment to be deprived of it through remediable ignorance. The physician who accepts such a policy clearly acts unethically, since duties to patients are disregarded without the patient's being made aware of the physician's dual role. The Code of Ethics of the American Society for Occupational Medicine requires physicians working in such settings to "avoid allowing medical judgment to be influenced by any conflict of interest" and "to accord highest priority to the health and safety of the individual in the work place." This implies that conflicts should be resolved in favor of individual patients, even if this is to the detriment of the company and the physician. Physicians accepting positions with dual responsibilities should be certain that their employers will allow them to abide by the ethical code. [The Code of Ethics of the American Society for Occupational Medicine. *Occupational Medicine* 1976; 8: cover.]

**4.9** **PUBLIC HEALTH**

Public health is the science and practice of preventing disease and promoting health in populations. As a science, it depends largely on epidemiology and, as a practice, is largely performed by governmental organizations, such as the Centers for Disease Control and local health departments. The traditional objectives were the control of communicable disease, the safety of the water and food supply, and response to natural disasters. More recently, public health has turned to broad educational efforts to enhance the health of the public by warning of health risks, informing about healthy life-styles, and encouraging preventive care, such as prenatal care. Many of the ethical issues of public health are matters of policy and are beyond the scope of this book. However, public health intersects with clinical care at several points. The protection of the public from communicable diseases, for example, conflicts with the medical duty of confidentiality. This is discussed at 4.2.3. Also, as "outcome studies" are applied to clinical decision-making and employed as guides for resource use, the general statistical data of epidemiology must be translated into the needs of particular patients. This is discussed at 4.3. One aspect of public health, the immunization of children, is a particular issue for pediatric ethics.

**4.9.1 P Immunization**

Vaccination is a major public health measure and is important to the health of individual children. The long effort by pediatricians to institute mandatory or universal immunization is threatened by changes in public health law which permit persons whose religious beliefs oppose such procedures to refuse vaccination and by the growing awareness of parents that vaccination has risks that could lead to serious and possibly uncompensated harm for their children. While this is distressing, the basic principle must be recalled: vaccination does put a child at some small risk of major harm to avoid a somewhat remote threat to its own health in order to contribute to the general safety of other children.

*COMMENT:*    When immunization is compulsory by law, the pediatrician does not obtain "informed consent" (with its counterpart, "informed dissent") from the parents. Rather, full information is given about the necessity for immunization and its risks. If immunization is not compulsory, the pediatrician must respect the parents' wishes, although efforts to educate and persuade are suitable. If parents refuse immunization against a serious disease of epidemic proportions, legal authorization should be sought. The problem of compensation for the harms due to immunization is a matter of social policy. Pediatric medicine should work to ensure the establishment of an equitable system for compensation of those who are involuntarily exposed to risks for the public good.

**4.10**                    **ETHICS COMMITTEES**
**AND ETHICS CONSULTATION**

In the usual course of the practice of medicine, important decisions are, and should be, made by the patient and physician together. Usually, outside parties have no right to partake in those decisions unless invited to do so by the principal parties. The growing complexity of the ethical issues in clinical care has stimulated the development of ethics committees and of ethics consultation. Ethics committees are established in health care institutions as advisory groups on policy and sometimes on cases that involve ethical issues. It is their responsibility to be familiar with the literature and methods of the field of bioethics and to make available to those who seek their counsel the best informed opinions about issues. Many judicial opinions have endorsed the idea of ethics committees as a means of resolving disputes before the participants are forced to the courts. Ethics consultation is modeled on the familiar practice of professional consultation: certain persons who have training in the field of bioethics are available to practitioners, and sometimes to patients, to review the facts of a particular case and offer informed and prudent counsel suited to the case.

Increasing attention to ethics by hospital accrediting agencies has renewed interest in the proper authority, scope, and methods of ethics consultation and committees. The President's Commission on Ethical Problems in Medicine considered three functions of ethics committees: education, policy development, and case consultation. The Federal Patient Self-Determination Act of 1991 stimulated community educational activities, often undertaken by ethics committees as well as professional organizations. In recent years many teaching hospitals and other health care institutions have employed individual ethics consultants or have authorized members of an ethics committee to offer case consultation. Some ethics committees develop institutional policies on matters such as DNAR or management of patients in a persistent vegetative state. Another recent development is the use of dispute resolution techniques like informal negotiation or mediation as an alternative to litigation when conflicts arise between patients or families and physicians. Ethics consultants and committees, risk managers, and legal counsel may collaborate to find informal solutions to value conflicts. For example, if physicians and parents disagree about the treatment plan for a severely and possibly terminally ill child, the dispute might be mediated by seeking an outside opinion from someone acceptable to physicians and parents. Even if physicians and parents fail to agree on everything, compromises might be achieved. If that fails, the parents have the option of transferring the child to a different institution. One general goal of an ethics program is to identify and manage ethics conflicts by seeking solutions rather than provoking litigation. Those problems that cannot be resolved by informal procedures may require formal legal resolution.

An effective ethics committee requires the following:

(a) Endorsement and support from the hospital administration and the medical and nursing staff. That support should include sufficient resources for the committee and consultants to function efficiently. The committee should be located clearly and appropriately in the institution's organizational chart, with designated lines of reporting.

(b) Members should be persons who are respected by their peers. They should meet regularly and keep records of their deliberations and of case consultations. Records should be maintained as confidential, according to the relevant laws.

(c) The committee should take measures to inform the staff of its existence and role and the procedures whereby it is contacted. Educational functions, such as occasional grand rounds or noon conferences, should be sponsored.

(d) Members and potential members should be given the opportunity and support to pursue education in medical ethics. Many educational opportunities are now available throughout the country.

(e) We recommend that committees and consultants review cases according to the method proposed in this book. [EB: "Clinical Ethics, Clinical Ethics Consultation, Institutional Ethics Committees," I, 399–412; Evaluation of case consultation in clinical ethics. *J Clin Ethics* 1996; 7(2):109–149; Cranford RE, Doudera AE. *Institutional Ethics Committees and Health Care Decision Making.* Ann Arbor: Health Administration Press, 1984; Hosford B, *Bioethics Committees: A Health Care Provider's Guide.* Rockville: Aspen, 1986; President's Commission for the Study of Ethical Problems in Medicine and Biomedical and Behavioral Research. *Deciding to Forego Life-Sustaining Treatment. A Report on the Ethical and Legal Issues in Treatment Decisions.* Washington, D.C.: Government Printing Office, 1983; Fletcher JC, Quist N, Jonsen AR, eds. *Ethics Consultation in Health Care.* Ann Arbor: Health Administration Press, 1989.]

**4.11**                                 **SUMMARY**

Clinical decisions are made in social, cultural, economic, legal, and educational contexts. All of these contexts generate certain rights and responsibilities. Clinicians have a primary ethical and legal responsibility to assure the well-being and dignity of their patients; and at the same time, they have other responsibilities that may, on occasion, conflict with their primary one. They must be aware of the extent of the just claims of other persons and institutions and take account of them to the extent compatible with their duties to their patients.

ISBN 0-07-033120-0

9 780070 331204

90000